*Handwritten notes:*
P108   www.oldwayspt.org/pyramids
veg pyramid

# Body
### *for*
# LIFE®
### *for Women*

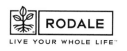

**RODALE**
LIVE YOUR WHOLE LIFE™

Every day our brands connect with and inspire millions of
people to live a life of the mind, body, spirit — a whole life.

# Body *for* LIFE *for Women*

## A WOMAN'S PLAN FOR PHYSICAL AND MENTAL TRANSFORMATION

### PAMELA PEEKE, MD, MPH, FACP
#### FOREWORD BY CINDY CRAWFORD

RODALE

© 2005 by Pamela Peeke, MD

Rodale Books may be purchased for business or promotional use or for special sales. For information, please write to: Special Markets Department, Rodale Inc., 733 Third Avenue, New York, NY 10017

Body-*for*-LIFE® is a registered trademark of Experimental and Applied Sciences, Inc. (EAS).

Printed in the United States of America
Rodale Inc. makes every effort to use acid-free ∞, recycled paper ♻.

Exercise photographs by Mitch Mandel/Rodale Images. Before and after photos provided by EAS.

**Library of Congress Cataloging-in-Publication Data**

Peeke, Pamela.
    Body-for-LIFE for women : a woman's plan for physical and mental transformation / Pamela Peeke.
        p.    cm.
    Includes index.
    ISBN-13 978–1–57954–601–4 hardcover
    ISBN-10 1–57954–601–3 hardcover
    ISBN-13 978–1–60529–828–3 paperback
    ISBN-10 1–60529–828–X paperback
    1. Women—Health and hygiene.   2. Women—Mental health.   3. Physical fitness
for women.   4. Weight loss.  I. Title.
RA778.P3167   2005
613'.04244—dc22                                          2004027374

Distributed to the trade by Macmillan

12  14  16  18  20  19  17  15  13  11 hardcover
2  4  6  8  10  9  7  5  3  1 paperback

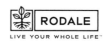

**We inspire and enable people to improve their lives and the world around them**
For more of our products visit **rodalestore.com** or call 1-800-848-4735

I dedicate this book to all of the women I have worked with, as well as the people who love them, who humble me with their stories of resilience in the face of adversity, and the tenacious ability to regroup when life's struggles seemed overwhelming. Their experiences confirmed my unwavering conviction that you can learn all you want about healthy eating and physical activity, but if you don't start first with the mind, you will never achieve your goal of lifelong wellness. They helped me create my Mind, Mouth, and Muscle triad, establishing a more holistic and integrative approach to caring for the mind and body. As I write these words, I recall so many women I have met over the years—an endless sea of feminine courage and tenacity.

I also dedicate this book to all of you who want to accept the challenge to push your feminine envelope and transform your life. All of you have the capacity to achieve your own optimal mind and body. In the words of Tommy Lasorda, "The difference between the impossible and the possible lies in a person's determination." It's that mind thing again.

So, to all of you, from the bottom of my heart, for your inspiration. As you start your journey, that's me on the sidelines, applauding your efforts and cheering you on with my enthusiastic, "Bravo! You go, girl!"

*Pam, you have always provided the inspiration, the encouragement, and the courage to deal with difficult times. With so many challenges—advanced cancer in my family, including my husband, my own breast cancer recurrence—it is easy to feel overwhelmed. I asked you for "magic," which would enable me to stuff the distress deep inside and focus on making the most of each precious day for my husband and me. Your advice was "Fill each day with as much joy and love as possible. Magic is found there, as well as the deeper peace you achieve as you embrace the belief that you're a marvelous whole of mind, body, and spirit, and that is your gift to the world." My Peeke Performer adventures with you—both the unforgettable post–September 11 New York City Marathon and the mountain hike to the summit of Aspen's Green Mountain in August 2003—have been simply transporting for mind, body, and spirit. Both those adventures allowed me to seize the opportunity just for a few days to leave chemotherapy behind, to breathe in every moment with love, to find the greatest imaginable joy in the beauty of nature, and to savor intensely a passion for living. Even now those moments of joy and wonder are crystal-clear memories for me. Is there any better way to live than so intensely in the moment, as we did?*

*I remember reaching the summit of the mountain and gazing at the unspeakable beauty of the vast panorama of mountaintops that surrounded me, amazed at my accomplishment. It was then that I suddenly realized that any worried thoughts about cancer were gone. Instead I was filled with a peaceful calm as I became aware of the power of my body and the strength of my mind. I can do anything.*

—Betty Lawson, breast cancer survivor and Peeke Performer

# Contents

# Acknowledgments

Writing this book has been an extraordinary team effort. Getting off first base is always Amanda Urban's job. As my literary agent, I'm supremely thankful that she's been by my side calling the shots and being my greatest cheerleader. The Rodale contingent is an extraordinary group of women. Nothing happens without superb leadership, and in my case it showed up in full force with Tami Booth, vice president and editor-in-chief of Rodale's Women's Books. She believed in the book and threw her might behind it. Julia VanTine-Reichardt, a master of wordsmithing, was my writing buddy. There's a special place in heaven for Julia, whose second career became tracking me down as I wrote on trains and planes and in between seeing patients, lecturing medical students, and doing television and radio segments. She now knows more about me than I care to acknowledge. Suffice it to say, she's an artist par excellence, and I know our friendship will continue long after this book. Ruler of the word is my editor Mariska van Aalst. I break out in a "deadline" sweat when I hear her name. Her brilliance and tenacity made this book a reality. Bravo, Mariska.

From the original EAS Body-*for*-LIFE team, I am thankful first to EAS board member, Augie Nieto, the founder of and genius behind the Life Fitness corporation. A friend and colleague, Augie inspired me to change directions in my book writing and tackle the challenge of gender-specific health and wellness. He also taught me that in life "you have to do what you don't want to do, in order to do what you do want to do." Late at night pounding away on my computer keys, grinding out the text, his words were a comfort. I thank Monty Sharma as well as Steve Breen for their efforts guiding the book to completion and beyond. Northcastle Partner's chairman Charles Baird, along with partner Brent Knudson, helped me navigate the tedious times forging the collaboration between Rodale and EAS. Of course, meeting with Bill Phillips confirmed the importance of writing this book.

Throughout my life, I have been blessed by mentors, like Augie, who've helped to light the way. From the moment he asked me to speak for the World President's Organization, I knew that Ira Brind would be one as well. His kindness and words of wisdom have helped shape my professional life.

Needless to say, none of this would be possible without my own estrogen squad, headed by the inimitable Vinita Stone, my executive assistant. She knows where I am before I'm there. That's scary stuff. Queen of my calendar, protector of my time, Vini shared her own life stories with me as we worked side by side laboring over every aspect of the book's execution. Words cannot capture my heartfelt gratitude for Vini in my life. And throughout the writing process, my wondrous medical practice manager, Torné, made room for every patient. Torné is a wonder herself. Having removed 130 pounds 11 years ago and kept it off, she is the epitome of the transformation in this book. My patients at the Peeke Performance Center love to hear her explain how everyone who wants it bad enough can succeed. At my center, chief nutritionist Eva Rand provided me with expert reviews of text while my mental therapist, Sharon Frischett, shared her insights on gender-specific psychology.

I am eternally indebted to all of my patients who took the time to share their stories and personal insights. These priceless gifts will touch your soul.

In writing this book, I counted on the wisdom and expertise of so many of my friends and colleagues, including Vivian Pinn, M.D.; Amy Niles; Jim Hill, Ph.D.; Jon Peters, Ph.D.; George Chrousos, M.D.; Barbara Moore, Ph.D.; Barbara Rolls, Ph.D.; Miriam Nelson, Ph.D.; and Ken Cooper, M.D.

My dearest friends Linda Solheim, Nancy Hazleton, Kay Kirkpatrick, Art and Sheila Walsh, and Naomi Henderson provided emotional support. I maintained my own body for life at the gym under Eric Eckenrode's expert guidance. Finally, I thank my family for their patience and love. Throughout the entire project, Mark was ever present, keeping me centered, and nurturing me as only a soul mate can do. For all of this, I am greatly blessed.

# Real-World Proof

## Preface

*"If I could do it, any woman can. In fact, you'll come to see that there's nothing, nothing, you can't do, once you believe that you can."*

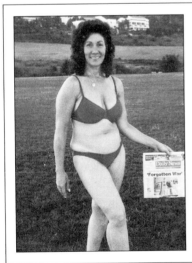 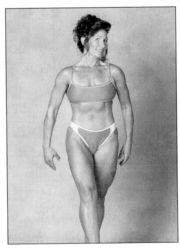 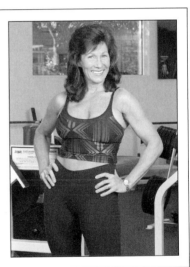

| Before | After | 4 Years Later |

**By Pamela Hickerson**

How does a 47-year-old woman who was just handed her divorce papers, with 30 pounds to lose and no self-esteem, turn her life around?

At that time in my life, I would have said, "Don't ask me." I had just walked away from a 10-year marriage to a handsome, successful lawyer. So saddened by my failure to please him, I even let him handle the divorce. I did not want anything. "All I wanted was your love," I had told him, which was the one thing he seemed unable to give.

It's not that he was a bad guy. We were just completely mismatched. During the entire marriage, I lived with a man who was never attracted to me, and my weight became a problem. Living in that loveless marriage, we shared an active social life with fascinating friends but not much else. I wanted children; he did not. We both spent most of our lives working on our careers, never on our relationship. I was depressed and very lonely. And, well, we all know what women do when they are depressed, lonely, bored, or angry, don't we? We eat, trying to satisfy that empty place inside. As I gained more weight, I felt less and less attractive.

After the divorce, I moved into a beat-up mobile home a couple of miles from the multimillion-dollar home overlooking the ocean in Malibu that we had shared together. I remember thinking about my former life, my career in TV production, and wondering, "I used to be a success—what happened?" Now my only comfort was a large pizza and a bottle of fine wine, which I could polish off while watching a movie at home. I still remember those late-night visits to the refrigerator—eating out of the gallon ice cream container one spoonful at a time, and why put the chocolate syrup on my ice cream when I could squirt it directly into my mouth? The same for whipped cream, so why not take the whole can to the couch?

At the time of the divorce, I was carrying 157 pounds on my 5-foot 6-inch body. Back in high school, I was a cheerleader and loved gymnastics. How did I get so out of touch with my body? How did I let myself get so fat? I'd tried to get into shape off and on, mostly to get my husband's attention and approval. I'd see a perfect body running on the beach and think, "If only I looked like her, he'd love me."

A funny game the mind plays on you. I was focused only on my exterior. It never occurred to me to think more deeply about the causes of my unhappiness. It's not surprising that I always sabotaged my attempts to lose weight.

And now I was alone. For the first 6 months after the divorce, I was in a very dark place. All I did was work and come home to my little mobile home and eat. I locked myself away and did not want to join the life of the living. I felt so depressed and defeated. I had made all the wrong choices in my life, and now, as I approached 50 years old, there seemed to be no hope for a happy future.

The one bright spot in my life was Paul, who had moved into the mobile home next to me. He was an unlikely friend—a guy, 10 years younger than me, and a really handsome Hawaiian who loved the ocean and surfed whenever he had the chance. He, too, had just gone through a difficult divorce and seemed to understand my pain. He helped me repair my mobile home, and in the process, we became dear friends. His children lived with him half the time, and when they were with him, we all played on the beach together. I adored them.

During this time, a girlfriend told me about the Challenge. She was one of *those* women—the ones who already have perfect bodies but think they're fat. She said to me, "Pam, I'm going to do this Body-*for*-LIFE. Do you want to do it with me?"

I had just turned 47 and felt adrift—no energy, no muscle tone, no spark for life. Up to this point, I had never finished anything I'd ever started. I needed something to *ignite* me. I needed this Challenge. I decided to give it all I had and not let anything get in my way.

A little embarrassed, I asked Paul if he would take my "before" picture. As he snapped away, he told me I looked great already, which made me feel a little better.

Then I got the pictures back. Yikes!

I was very disciplined with the diet part of the Challenge—yes, me, the emotional eater. I hit the gym at the same time every night, exactly when all the beautiful people in southern California work out to be seen and hook up with other beautiful people. I wore big, sloppy T-shirts and a baseball cap and put on my headset so I wouldn't have to talk to anyone. I really didn't care what anyone thought of me. I was there for myself.

I was ignored the first couple of weeks, but when others could see how determined and serious I was, they actually started to help me out and encourage me. The harder I worked out, the more respect I started to receive.

Despite my determination, the first month was tough. Every muscle in my body hurt. My soreness was overwhelming, but I loved it. I felt as if I was awakening again, and the soreness proved I was alive.

I didn't really see any changes until the 8th week—I never looked in the mirror. I remember that I was brushing my teeth, when I saw a muscle in my arm. There it was—a biceps. I said, "Wow, when did that happen?"

But just when you are making progress, life throws something your way. In week 8, I received devastating news: The man I loved most in this world, my father, had been diagnosed with prostate cancer. He had surgery, and I took him to his radiation and chemo treatments. At first, I thought I'd have to abandon the Challenge. But my father began to ask me if I'd done my workout that day. He loves me fat or skinny and did not want to take my efforts too seriously, in case I abandoned them. But he said, "I like you better when you are working out—you're in a better mood!"

When I mentioned quitting to Paul, he said, "How are you going to help your father if you can't help yourself? You need to be strong to help your dad be strong."

I think that was a turning point for me, understanding that I could help my father only if I first took care of myself. When I went to the gym that night, and from that point on, my workouts were transformed. I lifted heavier weights than ever before. I looked fear in the face—fear about my father, fear about my life—and conquered all my demons. Not even a sprained ankle in week 11 slowed me down.

Long story short—by week 12, I'd lost 26 pounds of pure fat and gained 6 pounds of pure muscle. I'd gone from 27 percent body fat to 13.9 percent and had dropped three dress sizes. Before, I'd struggled into size 11/12. Now I could slip into a size 5/6. I hardly recognized the person I had become.

While getting ready to take my "after" photos, I realized that the changes on the outside did not even begin to compare with the changes that had taken place on the inside. The walls I had put up around myself had come crashing down. I had proved something to myself: Life holds no barriers, only challenges.

The day after my pictures were taken, Paul and I went ocean kayaking. I was on cloud nine. I understood at last that the transformation is about much more than just improving your physical appearance; it's about taking control of your life. I was not afraid to go any-where, take on anything. I didn't just *feel* like a different person. I *was* a different person.

"You're a champion," Paul told me.

I said, "No, I'm not."

"Yes, you are," he replied. "Look up the word *champion* in the dictionary."

So I did. One definition said, "A person that is clearly superior or has the attributes of a winner." Hmmm, I could not argue with that. I felt that I had won back something infinitely precious: my life.

Another one was "An ardent defender or supporter of a cause or another person." I could not argue with that one, either. I'd learned to honor my body and the promises I made to myself, even as I was helping support my dad. I wasn't afraid anymore. I believed in myself again.

And yet another definition: "One who fights; a warrior." Every day I walked into that gym, with every drop of sweat and grunt of pain, I fought for myself because I knew, deep down, I was worth the fight. I realized that what made me a champion was my desire and passion and courage and faith that *I could do this*.

But really, my story has just begun. Soon after I finished the Challenge, Paul and I got married. We now live together in a mobile home we bought together on the beach in Malibu, just two coves down from where my ex-husband still lives. I've been blessed with the gift of his two adorable children in my life. My father's cancer is now in remission, and he and I have a company together. Not a day goes by when I don't appreciate having him with me on my new path. Paul has taught me to surf. We go kayaking together. We build sand castles. We love our life together.

Incredibly, my ex-husband and I are friends now. I think he is happy that I found someone. But I know that deep down he is still amazed at the shape I am in now. I heard this story from a friend of my ex's: A couple of months before Paul and I got married, I was attempting to surf, and my ex and a friend were on the beach, watching from a distance.

"Check out that woman on the board—she's pretty hot. Do you know who she is?" asked my ex.

"You're kidding, right?" his friend replied. "That's your ex. That's Pam."

And you know what? It *is* me. There's a scripture that I love, Isaiah 30:21, which reads, "And your own ears will hear a word behind you saying, this is the way, walk in it." I felt that I had found the way at last, and that I was in touch with my higher self.

That is really what the Challenge did for me—and if I could do it, any woman can. In fact, you'll come to see that there's nothing, *nothing*, you can't do, once you believe that you can.

Come on. Believe in yourself. Fight for yourself. Honor yourself. Accept the Challenge. Say yes.

# *Foreword*

## *By Cindy Crawford*

I've been a model since I was 17 years old, and unfortunately, I'm not one of those models who can eat anything they want and never work out (I quietly curse those girls, too). I had to choose a healthy lifestyle, to learn how to eat right—most of the time—and to exercise. And having to climb into a bikini in front of sometimes-critical fashion people at any time of year and in any kind of weather certainly keeps me motivated to consistently stay in shape.

Despite the barrage of wonder diets that guarantee quick weight loss by luring us to believe that if we eliminate this, control that, stop eating, or take a pill then we'll miraculously achieve our dream body, I pretty much maintain the health-and-fitness regimen that's worked for me since I was 22. Of course, different times in my life have brought about different challenges: losing baby weight, preparing for a *Playboy* shoot, or feeling especially good in my wedding dress. But I still believe that the most important and effective path to improved health, vitality, and weight loss is long-term, consistent motivation, which is what most diets are missing—and that's what Dr. Pam Peeke's book, *Body*-for-*LIFE for Women,* is all about. It's about change, about committing to a new way of living—one that will ensure a lifetime of self-esteem and confidence. It springs from a fundamental understanding of what works and what doesn't in both our minds and bodies.

In reading the personal success stories of women who made the commitment to change how they were living and, as a result, how they felt about themselves, I immediately thought of my mother. My mom always told me that it's easier to keep the weight off than to take it off. Unfortunately, this is something she learned the hard way. She was always struggling with 20 pounds, and I remember her starving herself or deciding to try a diet (one of which included eating six bananas in one day). Food was not her friend, and while it gave her comfort, the relationship wasn't easy. It was only when my mom committed to the Body-*for*-LIFE for Women program that she reclaimed her wellness. She even appeared to grow an inch as her posture improved, and her newfound dedication and restored confidence added a new dimension to our relationship as we talked about protein and carbs and compared exercise routines.

*Body*-for-*LIFE for Women* embraces women and all of our insecurities and weaknesses and then empowers us by giving us the information and tools to overcome them. The Body-*for*-LIFE for Women program emphasizes the importance of realizing life's stresses, no matter what they are or how big or small they are, and is a respectful and mindful motivational guide. The real-life success stories are not only proof of Dr. Pam Peeke's wisdom and understanding of women of every age, occupation, race, and size but also an inspiration to continue on a path of healthy living.

# The Breakthrough for Women

## Part 1

*"Optimism is the faith that leads to achievement. Nothing can be done without hope and confidence."*
—Helen Keller

We met on a fine autumn day in 2001. Then 48, Margaret, a talented editor who sat anxiously in my waiting room, was in full-throttle perimenopause. I led her to my office, offered her a seat in the Victorian armchair across from my desk, and asked why she'd come.

I had a pretty good idea.

She looked at me and tried to smile. Instead, her eyes welled with tears.

"I'm 5 feet 5 inches and 236 pounds. I wear a size 22. I'm disgusted with my body—and scared that I'm going to die."

Back then, studies had just begun to implicate excess inner abdominal fat—what I call Toxic Fat—as a risk factor for heart disease and diabetes, among other illnesses. Margaret was aware of these studies, and she had reason to worry. The workup I gave her that day said it all.

Fully 45 percent of her body was fat. Her fasting blood sugar, cholesterol, and blood pressure were all above normal. Her mother had both heart disease and diabetes, and

Margaret was following in her footsteps. She wanted to be there for her three children. She was having nightmares about losing it all.

I told her that to save her life, she had to change it. Then, together, we customized a new method of living that would work for her—a new way to eat, move her body, and manage the stress that was undermining her physical and emotional well-being.

Several months into her program, she left me a voice mail. Her husband, Richard, was ill. She'd be back as soon as the crisis was resolved. I sighed—I was concerned that she'd abandon all the positive changes she'd made. Who could blame her?

But 5 months later, there she was. In my waiting room. I'd walked right past her. You see, she'd really changed. The sad, defeated Margaret I'd met months before had been transformed into a smiling, serene-looking, and very fit woman.

Margaret told me that Richard had developed a life-threatening intestinal blockage and had had to spend weeks in the intensive care unit of a major medical center 60 miles from her home. She'd spent 4 months by his bedside.

I thought: This woman had the perfect excuse to let herself go—a sick husband, a boatload of stress. She could have stopped working out, started eating badly again.

Instead, she brought her own healthy meals to her husband's hospital room and left his side long enough each day to walk briskly around the hospital campus. She'd even gotten a short-term membership at a local gym to get in her weight lifting.

Margaret had removed 45 pounds. Her body fat was down 7 points. She'd lost 4 inches off her waist, and her fasting blood sugar and cholesterol were within normal limits. Her blood pressure was down, too.

"Awesome. Absolutely awesome," I said, giving her a hug. "How'd you do it?"

Smiling, Margaret said, "When my husband got sick, I wanted to crawl in bed and pull the covers over my head. I knew I had to stay strong—for him, for my family—but I didn't know how I was going to pull it off.

"One day as I was stressing out, this image of myself popped into my head. I was a woman warrior. I had the sword, the breastplate, the whole deal, and I was fighting for my husband's life."

Sounds very Xena, right? But that image gave her focus. Purpose. Every time she walked, lifted weights, chose to fuel her body with good, healthy food, she was staying strong. For him, and for her children.

But somewhere along the line, Margaret started getting stronger not just for them but for herself.

"I felt powerful," Margaret said. "My muscles were stronger. My mind was clearer. By the time my husband had recovered, I felt like I'd been reborn."

Right then, I got it. This woman had cracked the code. She'd stayed with her program because she'd decided, consciously or not, to *fight for her own life as fiercely as she'd fought for her husband's.*

And that, girlfriends, is the core of *Body-for-LIFE for Women.*

## THE SEARCH FOR A WOMAN'S FORMULA

In my first book, *Fight Fat after Forty,* I helped introduce the world to the stress–fat connection with the aim of helping women prevent what I called Toxic Fat, the stubborn fat inside your belly that accumulates when stress is out of control and that has been linked to many deadly chronic diseases.

Since the publication of that book, we know more than ever before about women's health. The bad news: Women's health has gotten worse! Over 30 percent of women carry at least 50 pounds more than recommended for optimal health. And, frighteningly, their daughters are becoming so sedentary and overweight that they risk becoming the first generation not to live as long as their parents. These changes only further steeled my resolve to develop a solution that would help women live longer, healthier lives. I'd heard of the book *Body-for-LIFE,* of course—was there anyone left on the planet who hadn't heard of this program for physical and mental transformation?—but when I hatched the plan for my second book, I hadn't yet read it. One afternoon, I picked up *Body-for-LIFE,* sat down, and read it cover to cover.

And it got me thinking. I'd treated lots of women over the years. They had had babies, got PMS every month, were going through perimenopause, or were well past menopause. Normal woman things. And though many got very fit during our work together, many struggled with creating the time and the emotional space for themselves to change their bodies the way they wanted to.

I knew from my practice that the most successful plan for today's women would factor in the realities of a woman's whole life—the full-time job, the endless caregiving, the stress that comes with trying to do it all. It would also recognize the importance of specific nutrients women need for optimal health, like calcium, iron, and folic acid. It would certainly need to accommodate the fluctuations in mood, energy, and appetite that happen around the time of a woman's period or during peri-menopause. And, most clearly of all, it would address the issues of emotional eating and poor body image—issues with which many women struggle on a daily basis.

I liked the idea of achieving a fit, healthy body "for life," and how the program revolved around a personal 12-week Challenge. I knew from my work with my patients that the very word *challenge* suggested hope, potential, empowerment. When you accept a challenge, you step up to the plate and give it your all. Roll up your sleeves, so to speak, and get to work. And when the challenge is met, you get to savor the rewards of your efforts. Just for fun, I began to play with the program—to modify it to a woman's unique physical and emotional makeup. And, as life would have it, I met Bill Phillips, the author of the original *Body*-for-*LIFE*, in Washington, D.C., on a snowy night in January 2004. We talked for hours, and it was clear that we both wanted to help people achieve their optimal mind and body, each from our own uniquely male and female points of view. That's when I resolved to bring the Body-*for*-LIFE program to a wider audience of women and give them the opportunity to achieve their own physical and mental transformation.

The result? This mind/body program of transformation for women, which synthesizes the newest science; my expertise in the fields of nutrition, stress, and metabolism; and my experience in helping thousands of women revitalize their health and their lives. Body-*for*-LIFE for Women is a refinement of the original Body-*for*-LIFE program, a holistic, integrated plan for healthier living that incorporates information about nutrition, exercise, and stress management specifically chosen to help women achieve their Body-*for*-LIFE.

## VIVE LA DIFFÉRENCE!

The women I work with are of all ages, weights, and fitness levels. Body-*for*-LIFE for Women is working for them, and I believe it will work for you, too. This program factors in elements—such as age and hormonal levels—that have a significant impact on a woman's body composition, weight, and fitness level. And there's a blueprint for using this program *for life*. Here's how the program will help you achieve optimal health.

**It's based on scientific breakthroughs in two of the hottest fields of research.** The first is gender-specific medicine, the science of how gender impacts the diagnosis and treatment of disease. This book focuses on the latest research in nutrition and fitness that has been conducted on women, rather than on men.

The second hot area of research is body composition (body comp for short), the proportions of fat, muscle, and bone that make up total body weight. By using this measure as its foundation, Body-*for*-LIFE for Women gives women a whole new paradigm for health and disease prevention. The scale weight is but one data byte. Now we focus on the quality of a woman's weight, not just the quantity. As my patient Marilyn once said, "Dr. Peeke, if I lost my keys, I'd want to find them. I haven't lost 63 pounds. I've *removed* them." So we no longer talk about weight "loss" but about *weight removal*.

**It's holistic.** With Body-*for*-LIFE for Women, the password is *fitness*—mental as well as physical. It's about having a sound mind in a sound body, and about achieving a balance between caring for the people you love and caring for yourself. In this paradigm, Mind always affects Body and vice versa, and it's the synergy between the two that creates health and fitness.

**It redefines the healthy female body.** With Body-*for*-LIFE for Women, the only standard you meet is based on you. If you're over 40, don't count on its helping you to squeeze into size zero jeans. But do expect a more lasting reward: a strong body that allows you to do the stuff you need—and want—to do without breaking down on you. It encourages you to embrace and optimize your mental and physical strengths by challenging you to be the very best you can be.

**It's woman-proof.** I've treated thousands of women, and not one of them was derailed by laziness or lack of willpower. No, they were done in by uniquely female traits.

The first: caregiving with no limits or boundaries. While women are busy making everyone else's life a little easier, their bodies and minds go to hell. As my patient Naomi once said, "I kept spending body dollars taking care of everyone else and forgetting about me!"

## Birthdays Don't Count, Hormonal Milestones Do

The average woman born in 1900 lived to be 48. Unbelievable. Some of us are still changing Pampers at that age! Though we're living longer now, we've always outlived men. The average woman now lives 79.5 years; the average man, 74.

Women live longer than men for a multitude of reasons—biological, behavioral, social, psychological. But these days, chronological age is only a tiny piece of the story. Thanks to medical breakthroughs, better nutrition, more physical activity, and a decline in smoking, the rate of disabilities among older people has dropped dramatically. Many of my perimenopausal or menopausal patients are running marathons or climbing mountains at 50-plus.

Body-*for*-LIFE for Women takes the original Body-*for*-LIFE program one step deeper, to incorporate a groundbreaking view of female health. Instead of fixating on chronological age, we'll talk in terms of our Hormonal Milestones. In this book, you'll learn how to optimize your health and your body's physical fitness during each of your Hormonal Milestones:

• Milestone 1: Menstruation to First Pregnancy

• Milestone 2: The Reproductive Years

• Milestone 3: Perimenopause

• Milestone 4: Beyond Menopause

Each Milestone represents a significant shift in a woman's hormonal makeup, and each has dramatic implications for her health. For example, in the first Milestone, the surge of estrogen and other female hormones affects our hearts, our bones, our fat stores, and even our emotions. In many ways, Milestone 4 is the mirror image of Milestone 1; the decline of these hormones—whether sudden or gradual—reframes our approach to physical and emotional well-being.

In part 2, you'll learn more about your Hormonal Milestones and how each impacts your body. Whether you're in Milestone 1 or beyond, you'll learn tactics that will help you reach your optimal level of health and fitness for this time of your life, which will set the stage for good health in the next, and the next, and the next.

The second: rumination, or obsessing about something without doing anything about it. Women rarely "just do it." For us, it's usually "just obsess about it." Well, that's about to end. No more agonizing that you're too fat to be seen in a gym. No more putting off your walks until you find a tracksuit that agrees with your skin tone. You already know what to do. Body-*for*-LIFE for Women shows you how to get it done.

**It is truly for life.** The core of Body-*for*-LIFE for Women centers on what happens during a specific 12-week Challenge. Each Challenge segment is part of an ongoing series of personal challenges—in which you're either shedding or maintaining weight—that you cycle through for the rest of your life. Whether it's pregnancy, illness, surgery, serious stress—or anything that causes you to regain the weight you've already removed—you'll have the tools to regroup and stay mentally and physically fit. (And who knows? Maybe you'll even be inspired to enter the EAS Body-*for*-LIFE Challenge contest (www.bodyforlife.com) and also have a chance at winning some cold, hard cash.)

So far, so good? Good. But there's a lot more to this program. Let's drill a little deeper.

## THE WINNING FORMULA: MIND-MOUTH-MUSCLE

Body-*for*-LIFE for Women uses a unique and integrative template for fitness that I call the Mind-Mouth-Muscle Formula—MMM for short. It's a woman's blueprint for being and staying physically and mentally fit at every stage of her life, despite her endless caregiving and her unique stressors. Using MMM to guide your Challenge is the best way I've ever seen for women to achieve their fittest, healthiest body, regardless of their age, health, or physical condition.

The MMM Formula encompasses a woman's . . .

• Attitude about balancing and managing the stresses of her life while caring for and honoring her mind and body (Mind)

• Way of nourishing herself to optimize her body composition and health (Mouth)

• Use of specific physical activity to attain and sustain her optimal body comp and performance (Muscle)

In the Mind: The 10 Body-*for*-LIFE for Women Power Mind Principles component, you'll learn how to navigate life's stresses in such a way that you won't keep falling off your own daily radar screen. The Mind component also helps you develop your own Motivational Target—a way of thinking that keeps you on track, no matter how tough your day can be. You'll also learn the 10 Power Mind Principles, which will serve as the foundation upon which you will achieve your Mouth and Muscle objectives.

In the Mouth: The Body-*for*-LIFE for Women Eating Method part of the formula, I'll teach you how to fuel yourself to get leaner and optimize your female body comp. I'll explain how striving only to "lose" weight is a dead end, and that your bones and muscles need to be fed appropriately while you shed health-threatening fat.

In the Muscle: The Body-*for*-LIFE for Women Training Method component, I'll show you how to perform the bottom-line amount of physical activity to achieve your personal-best body comp. You'll learn that the new message is not time (how long you exercise) but *intensity* (how hard you exercise). Pulling the whole program together, I'll show you how to defeat a woman's biggest fitness obstacle: her own lack of faith in herself.

The best part about the MMM Formula is that it helps the Body-*for*-LIFE program fit every woman. You define your own Challenge for yourself. You can use the program as is, tweak it slightly, or completely customize it to fit your unique lifestyle, temperament, and preferences.

## TROUBLESHOOTING MENTAL SPEED BUMPS

Of course, making changes is hard, and we all sometimes fight the fact that having a fit, healthy body takes effort and commitment. Believe me, I know—I'm fighting the good fight right along with you! It's all about being honest and realistic about the level of discomfort you're willing to experience to achieve the reward you want. Because I know it so well, I can map out the process by which we achieve this acceptance or abandon the fight. This "map" can help illuminate the process of achieving this acceptance.

**Step 1: Starting the journey.** Divine inspiration doesn't start the process. You do. Brushing aside your usual tendency to ruminate, you make the basic lifestyle changes—the walk after dinner rather than reruns, the apple instead of the doughnut.

At some point, life hits and you face tougher challenges. Stress. Boredom. Impatience. Depression. Frustration. This is where the talk meets the walk. You were willing to pay a certain price to remove your first pounds and ratchet up your fitness level. Now the "price" of a fit and healthy body is higher. Are you willing to pay? Or, if life is tough now, can you practice "treading weight," or maintaining the weight removal you've already accomplished?

**Step 2: Pushing the denial envelope.** You resist. You engage in little-kid "I don't wannas." You think there must be a way of working around the MMM rules. You say to yourself, "It's just a bag of chips" or "I hate to exercise." The result? The fat doesn't budge.

**Step 3: Should I or should I not?** That's what you'll say when you see a plate of buffalo wings in front of you or your walking shoes at the porch door. But are brushing your teeth and combing your hair ever up for discussion? Of course not. Neither should paying attention to your eating and doing physical activity. At this point, you're still doing the Great Debate, when you should just do it!

**Step 4: Connecting the dots.** Frustrated by a lack of results, you're banging your head against the wall, fighting the changes you must make. Then one day, the veil lifts and you see the consequences of your actions—or lack of action. You see cause and effect. No physical activity, no strength and endurance. No paying attention to eating, no weight removal. You connect the dots. You know that what you eat and what activity you do creates the body you have—and there's no getting around it.

Once you see this, you've arrived at a state of acceptance. There are two kinds of acceptance—one good, one not so good—and you will choose one or the other.

**Step 5: Resignation versus acceptance.** The first type of acceptance is *resigned* acceptance, when you accept that you're not willing to do what it takes to ensure your physical and mental well-being. We become resigned to being overweight and unhealthy and miserable. Then your mind goes into la-la land and denies the reality: You have a body. We've all been there, and it's not a pretty place.

The second type of acceptance is *humble, realistic* acceptance, in which you choose to move forward and accept that you must work for a fit, healthy body. You see the price and you're willing to pay it. You no longer fight this fact; you embrace it. Heck, you run with it!

Even if you're not quite there yet, press on. You're about to hear some amazing stories. The Body-*for*-LIFE for Women program will help you connect those dots so you can humbly accept the work. You'll have the precise plan to peel off that Toxic Fat and reveal a fitter, stronger, and more powerful you.

By the way, I encourage you to push the denial envelope. Every woman goes through good times of positive acceptance, and tougher times when she temporarily throws in the towel. When we were toddlers, we pushed it by touching the hot stove even though our mothers said not to. But we learned not to touch it again. Learning happens by pushing the envelope. I say, "Bring it on!" because it leads to transformation, and I'm all for that.

I also encourage you to have a lifetime of "successful relapse." Life happens, and you're bound to have times that result in personal turmoil, weight gain, and lack of fitness. But the key to successful relapse is to learn something that you can apply to your health and fitness journey. That's what Naomi, one of my patients, did.

A successful businesswoman, Naomi had come to me because her weight had begun to affect her physical and emotional well-being. After a period of fighting the changes she knew she needed to make to have a healthier body and mind, something clicked and she finally "got it." I'll let her tell her own story in her own words.

*At 37, I left corporate America and started my own business. I worked like a dog—100- to 120-hour weeks. I traveled 17 days out of every month. This went on for years.*

*As the business grew, so did I. I ate dinner at 10:30 P.M. and went to bed at 1:00 A.M. I got up at 5:00 A.M. and ate a huge breakfast, then later a big lunch, multiple snacks, and that late dinner. My only exercise was to lift suitcases over my head and push them into the overhead bin of a plane. I'm 5 feet 6 inches, and I blimped up from 130 pounds in my forties to over 200 pounds when I hit 50, in 1994.*

*In 1995, I took a yearlong sabbatical to see what retirement might be like, to write, and to work on myself and my body.*

*Just around that time, I saw an article about the work Dr. Peeke was doing with overweight men and women. There was a picture of Dr. Peeke next to a big man on a treadmill. His story sounded like mine: "All my energy goes into running my business. I don't eat right—late meals with clients—don't exercise."*

*I said, "Bingo! I need to see this doctor."*

*Dr. Peeke suggested that I begin my Challenge slowly. So I bought a treadmill. My plan was to walk every day. When I started, I could do only 5 minutes. I'd have to get off and lie down to catch my breath.*

*I did that for weeks. I would be so out of breath, and my knees hurt so bad. It was torture. But in my weekly visits with Pam (which included the occasional "walk and talk"), she convinced me I could improve.*

*Soon I was able to walk 7 minutes, then 10, then 20. After about 10 months, I could walk 45 minutes without a break. I also added weights to my program. I began to remove fat and build muscle.*

*During this time, I used the MMM Formula Dr. Peeke had taught me. Well, sort of. I did the cardio but not the lifting. I avoided the minibars in my hotel rooms but "forgot" to watch my portions. And although I knew full well what I needed to do to stay healthy, I fought it. I felt resentful that I had yet one more thing to do, one more burden to drag around with me.*

*Eventually, I noticed a pattern: When I didn't control my anger and resentment, I'd regain a few pounds or my progress would stall. When I told myself, "Just do it," and focused on working the program, I was rewarded. My energy went up, I slept better, the extra pounds slipped away, I felt stronger and more confident. On the day I noticed this, I thought to myself, "Why am I fighting something that's so right, that works so well for me?"*

*As soon as I asked that, I got it. The Click. I stopped fighting. The key was humble acceptance. When I achieved it, I felt a sense of peace and an end to my conflict and resentment about taking care of myself. Then and there, I pledged to transform my prior negative attitude into energy—energy spent on implementing the MMM Formula every day. Some days were better than others, of course, but I now fully acknowledge that I have to pay the price to feel this good. Every day, I accept that I am willing to pay that price.*

*Over a 3-year period, I removed 40 pounds. I still work 80-plus-hour weeks (my company, my choice), so I've learned to force-fit exercise into my life. I have a plan I call "doing my 21s," which is 21 minutes or 42 minutes or 63 minutes of exercise, whatever I can squeeze in. Sometimes I have to jog in place in my hotel room at 11:30 at night, but I get it in.*

*I also wear a pedometer everywhere I go and strive for 10,000 steps a day, minimum. I've ramped up my walking routine to include hill training, both on the treadmill and on real trails.*

*I get to the gym to lift weights once or twice a week and walk a minimum of 2 miles four to six times a week. In 2001, I joined Dr. Peeke and became a Peeke Performer by walking the New York City Marathon in 9 hours, 9 minutes, 52 seconds. That was the hardest thing I've ever done.*

*In 2004, I spent my 60th birthday on a weeklong hiking trip in Killington, Vermont. My goal is to live to be 100-plus and to have a body that will make that journey without a walker, cane, crutch, or wheelchair. On my 100th birthday, I want to be striding down a trail, swinging my arms and listening to jazz on my headset. That's the picture I hold in my mind when I want to make an excuse for why I don't have time to walk.*

For years, Naomi pushed her denial envelope. At some point, tired beyond belief and fed up with the same vicious cycle, Naomi connected the dots—click! *She got it.* Once she'd humbly accepted the price she was willing to pay to save her life, she felt a new sensation: peace. Her "Should I, or should I not?" was replaced by "When and how will I take that walk?" No more inner conflict. The war was over, and the victory was hers.

## THE BODY-*FOR*-LIFE FOR WOMEN PLEDGE

I promise that the Body-*for*-LIFE for Women program—which is supported by the latest research conducted exclusively on women—can help you get the fit, attractive, and healthy body that you've yearned for, and can help you optimize your body throughout your life. That is, if you're willing to move a little more, eat a little better, and make those subtle shifts that will increase your resilience in the face of chronic stress.

If you have that resolve, I promise you that you can have an optimal body. *Your* optimal body, not a fitness model's. You can keep fat at bay and hold on to lean, strong, calorie-burning muscle for the rest of your life.

Now I'd like you to take the Body-*for*-LIFE for Women Pledge:

*I will give to myself as I give to others.*
*I will value my health as I value the health of my loved ones.*
*I won't ask, "Should I or shouldn't I?" about matters of self-care.*
*I will just do it.*
*I humbly accept that I must work to be the best me I can be.*
*I will choose to work for myself, rather than abandon myself.*
*I will embrace adversity as an opportunity to test my mental and physical strength.*

If you make and honor this pledge, your physical and emotional health will take a dramatic turn for the better. I think you'll find life a whole lot more joyful and fulfilling, too. Because the truth is, you're here to do more than care for your family, or your job, as important and fulfilling as they may be. *Self* is not a four-letter word. You're here to experience life, to learn from all its uncertainties, adventures, joys, and dark patches. And at the end of the day, you are the only one who can give your life meaning.

Caring for ourselves doesn't come easily to women, but you can learn to do it—and see the value in it. As a scientist, a medical doctor, and a woman who's right there in the trenches with you, I invite you to try Body-*for*-LIFE for Women. To realign your mind with your body. To reconcile your physical health with your emotional well-being. To reclaim your Body-*for*-LIFE.

## LAUNCHING YOUR BODY-*FOR*-LIFE PLAN

To ensure your success, it is best to start the program with a solid foundation. That's why I suggest that before you so much as put on a gym sock or grill a chicken breast, you read the entire book from beginning to end.

Body-*for*-LIFE is an *integrative* program—all facets of the Mind-Mouth-Muscle Formula work better with the others in place. For example, part 2 of this book explores the unique differences in physiology between women and men. Part 2 lays the groundwork for part 3, Mind: The 10 Body-*for*-LIFE for Women Power Mind Principles, which gets you thinking about the motivation, or motivations, for your transformation; part 4, Mouth: The Body-*for*-LIFE for Women Eating Method; and part 5, Muscle: The Body-*for*-LIFE for Women Training Method. You'll discover how each piece of the program will help you achieve your goals, whether you choose to start with a Weight Removal Segment, or you want to "tread weight" with a Maintenance Segment. No matter where you begin, success starts with a positive attitude. To work the Mouth and Muscle Formulas, you have to have the Mind stuff down.

As you read, feel free to skim over the parts that are really easy for you. For example, if you've always been an athlete, the Muscle section will be familiar and friendly territory. Concentrate on the areas that are more challenging. For most of us, that would be the Mind section. Many women make a second career out of creating mental speed bumps to complicate their self-care journey. Once you understand our unique psychological tendencies, it's easier to see how to stay the course on your nutrition and physical fitness.

Once you've read, you can decide how you'd like to start your program. If you wish, you can go full throttle from day 1, integrating all three parts of the Mind-Mouth-Muscle Formula into your life. But you can also work on one or two parts of the program at a time. If you want to start eating more healthfully (Mouth) before you start working out (Muscle), fine by me. Or if you want to incorporate walking into your life first and then address weight lifting, fabulous. Whether you start all three components of the program from day 1 or phase them in, be kind to yourself. I never want to hear that P word—*perfect*—cross your lips. "I wasn't perfect!" Well, terrific. Your goal is not to be perfect. It's to be human and do the best you can within the limitations and constraints of your life.

Finally, I know you'll get stoked by the real-life success stories, which start on page 229. I hope these women inspire you as they describe how they were the instruments of their own transformations. You'll see their pictures as they began their Challenge, as well as pictures that give you a sense of how they feel about their bodies today, years later. All the women pictured in this book began their personal challenges by entering the 12-week, EAS Body-*for*-LIFE Challenge (see www.bodyforlife.com for details), most likely integrating Mouth and Muscle from day 1. But it is their long-term fitness that proves that *success is the achievement of a fit mind and body that can be sustained for life.* Dropping 20 pounds and gaining it right back is not success. Doing it right, and maintaining that change, is. Their stories will prove to you that this program really can transform you, and that the changes you make—both in your body and in your head—really are *for life.*

So hop to it, girlfriends. No rumination, no second thoughts. No doubts. Just pure, self-empowering action.

## SHE CAME OUT OF HIDING—BODY AND SOUL

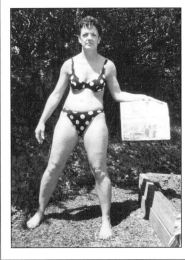 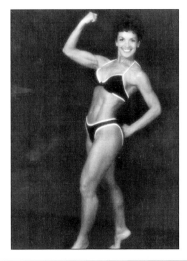 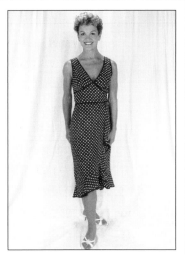

Before                                    After                              5 Years Later

The desire to change her life crept up on 52-year-old Pat Green, a real estate agent in Watsonville, California. "I was busy with my career, family, and community work but wasn't taking any time to take care of Pat. I was only 15 or 20 pounds over-weight, but I was miserably out of shape and out of energy."

One day, Pat caught a side view of herself in a plate-glass window and thought, "Whoa. How did this happen?" So she went home and stripped down in front of the full-length mirror in her bedroom. "I looked awful!" she remembers. "My hips had developed extra padding, my legs were chubby, and my waist had hidden beneath rolls of flab. I had no muscle definition. As I got dressed again, sucking in to close the buttons on my jeans, I thought, 'Well, metabolism slows down after 40, right?'"

But this explanation just didn't work for Pat. She was ready to change. "I hid my body with oversize clothing, and my sadness at being tired and out of shape behind a smile. I didn't want to hide anymore."

Pat had heard about the Body-*for*-LIFE program through her younger sister, who had just completed the Challenge herself and had removed a bunch of weight. "I thought the Body-*for*-LIFE Challenge was too good to be true, but I decided to give it a try."

Pat expected that it would take time to remove her excess pounds, boost her energy, and recapture her positive spirit. But only a few weeks into the program, she was bursting with energy, and stress just seemed to roll off her back.

At the end of 12 weeks, Pat had removed 15 pounds, and her body fat was cut in half, to 10 percent. She's sustained her healthier weight for more than 5 years now. And since she's learned to take time for herself on a regular basis, her life is immeasurably better.

"My three grown children and I enjoy walking and doing 10-K races, and we recently went skydiving at 18,000 feet. My renewed self-confidence tells me that I can do anything." Pat also got so involved with her aerobics classes that she now teaches five classes a week.

"I still keep my 'before,' 'fat' picture of myself in my gym bag and pull it out when someone doesn't believe my 'before' story. Sometimes when I pass a mirror and catch a glimpse of myself, I expect to see an overweight and unhealthy woman. Instead, I see a happy, healthy woman. That woman is me!"

## SHE CONQUERED CHRONIC PAIN AND REGAINED HER WAISTLINE

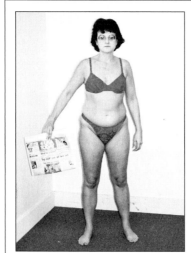 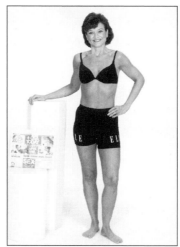 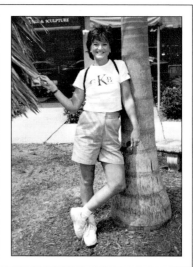

| Before | After | 5 Years Later |

At age 41, Jenifer Meyer, a resort sales manager from Huron, Ohio, was supposed to be in the prime of her life. But that was far from her reality.

"I was losing my 9-year battle with fibromyalgia. Each morning, I woke to more pain and depression. I couldn't do the simplest chores. I went from doctor to doctor, searched for help in books. Nothing helped, and everything hurt—I'd lived with chronic pain for years. But most of all, I was disgusted with my body—it was soft and fat from lack of exercise. I had to get a grip on my life."

Then her life took a turn for the better. A local gym offered a discount rate to the resort Jenifer worked at, which sparked her interest in exercise. But the turning point was when she read about the Body-*for*-LIFE Challenge in a magazine, 3 months after she'd begun working out. "I couldn't stop thinking about the possibility of overcoming my pain and regaining my life. But could I handle weight lifting? That was my greatest fear."

But Jenifer persevered, getting on the stationary bike or elliptical trainer each evening after work, and a trainer at the gym demonstrated the proper form and technique for the strength-training exercises. "I never thought I'd be able to lift weights—doing household chores was difficult for me. But I started out with light weights, and my strength slowly began to grow. The first 4 weeks were tough, but my pain was different. It was pain from sore muscles, not like the pain I'd had for the past 9 years, and not anywhere as intense as I was used to."

By the end of 12 weeks, the pain was completely gone. She was benching her own weight, and her energy was through the roof. "It was as if I'd put up a brick wall of muscle between me and the pain I had lived with for so many years." In 12 weeks, she removed 34 pounds of fat, gained 7 pounds of lean muscle, and reduced her waistline from 31 to 25 inches.

Jenifer has regained her edge on life and looks great. "But more important, I feel great. The Body-*for*-LIFE program isn't just a physical transformation—it's a mental transformation as well. You get reacquainted with yourself all over again. The 12-week Challenge forces you to reach down deep within yourself. My reward is strength—not just physical strength but mental strength. I've gained so much—self-confidence, self-esteem, self-respect."

## AT 95, SHE'S STILL GOT IT

When Edith Odoms, a retired schoolteacher from Walla Walla, Washington, first heard about Body-*for*-LIFE, she was 89 years old and had had two strokes. She was also confined to a wheelchair, having broken her hip after slipping on an ice-slicked sidewalk. Despite these obstacles, she was determined to get out of her wheelchair and heal her body.

It was her 51-year-old daughter, MaryAnn, who told her about the Body-*for*-LIFE

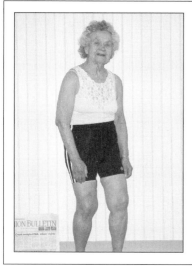 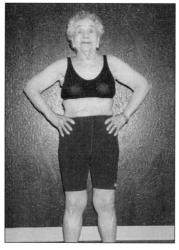 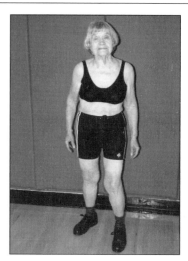

Before                          After                          6 Years Later

program and the Challenge; MaryAnn had heard about it from her own daughter. "My 90th birthday was coming up, and I asked my daughter if she thought the program could help me. When she said yes, I didn't give it a second thought."

Although Edith was determined to succeed, the program proved difficult for her at first. With her daughter's help, she lifted weights three times a week—from her wheelchair. "The improvements came little by little, but I was excited about each one." In just weeks, she was ready to rise from her wheelchair. "One day, I just got up out of it—slowly, but I did it." She began to walk, at first for just minutes at a time. She walked and rested, walked and rested. When she started, it took her 35 minutes to walk 1 mile; in month 2, she did it in 23 minutes. Soon she was walking 3 miles a day. Her physical health and mental outlook continued to improve.

Now 95, Edith is physically active almost every day—she takes a martial arts class, participates in a seniors' fitness class, and strength-trains three times a week. She ascends and descends stairs on her own, rises from chairs, and is able to get into and out of the car and tub. Her diet is still healthy, too—plenty of fresh fruits and veggies and lean protein. "I gave myself the gift of a whole, healthy body."

Edith says she'll never slow down. "I tell myself that if I slow down, there's another wheelchair waiting for me. My goal is to go on and never give up."

# The Measure of a Woman: From Body Comp to Hormonal Milestones

## Part 2

*"A woman is like a tea bag—you never know how strong she is until she gets in hot water."*

—Eleanor Roosevelt

As I was writing *Fight Fat after Forty,* gender-specific medicine—the science of how gender influences both health and disease—was in the very early stages of development. But just after my book was published, the field exploded. We now know that gender exerts a significant influence on mental and physical health. Thankfully, researchers now include women in their medical studies, and more and more physicians tailor their treatment to the unique characteristics of the female gender.

The Body-*for*-LIFE for Women plan takes full advantage of this burgeoning field of research. By using these new findings to customize the program to your specific physiology, you'll not only get the results you want on the outside—better girth control, improved muscle tone, a leaner, longer appearance—but also reap the health benefits on the inside, now and for years to come.

To appreciate how truly revolutionary this approach is, you have to remember that much of the health information still taken as gospel stems from research conducted entirely on—you guessed it—men.

It wasn't until 1990, the year before I started at the National Institutes of Health (NIH), that Bernadine Healy, M.D.—the first female director of the NIH—established the Office of Women's Research (OWR) and appointed my wonderful friend Vivian Pinn, M.D., as its director. And it's only since the creation of the OWR that women have been included in medical studies—in large part because, to be perfectly honest with you, women fought for it.

Since then, gender-specific medicine has taught researchers to appreciate that the male and the female bodies have unique strengths and vulnerabilities. As this relatively new field of medicine has evolved, amazing data has emerged, and some of the most striking discoveries have had significant implications for women's health.

Think about this:

• More women than men die each year from heart disease. Moreover, 39 percent of women die within a few weeks of their first heart attack, compared with 31 percent of men.

• Compared with nondiabetic women, women with diabetes have six times the risk of heart disease. By contrast, diabetic men have only twice the risk of heart disease as do nondiabetic men.

• Women are vulnerable to potentially fatal heart arrhythmias—deviations from normal heartbeat rhythms—when they take some of the same drugs that stabilize heart rhythms in men.

• The risk of lung cancer among women smokers is double that of men who smoke.

• Women are more prone to anxiety and panic than men are. It's now known that changing levels of reproductive hormones throughout our lives can affect our mood as well as our response to some antidepressants.

• Inactive women over 40 lose muscle mass twice as fast as inactive men do.

• Women secrete less of the brain chemical serotonin than men do, making them more vulnerable to depression, mood disorders, and overeating (especially carbs) under stress.

In light of the myriad ways we differ from men—not only biologically but in how we think about our eating, our exercise, and especially our emotions—it's important to understand how these differences manifest in our lifelong health. After all, when you undergo the Body-*for*-LIFE transformation, you're not just working toward that fitting-into-the-killer-jeans moment. You're saving your own life. By examining these key differences in our bodies in the following text, and how they change and develop over the course of our lives, I'm hoping to deliver the almighty kick in the ovaries that will help you make changes, take control, and truly reclaim your Body-*for*-LIFE.

## FAT, MUSCLE, AND GENDER

Gender-specific medicine has proven what virtually every woman over 35 has suspected: Gender has a significant influence on body fat and weight gain. Ever wonder why your partner sheds weight faster and more easily than you do? Of course you

---

**Warning! Warning! "Fat Gene" Alert!**

Does Mom or Dad, or their side of the family, tend to be on the heavy side? Have you always been heavy? If so, here's a big heads-up: You may harbor the so-called obesity (*ob*) gene. This means that you may have a propensity to store fat, even if you haven't been overweight up till now.

Why? Because the debut of each Milestone presents an opportunity for the *ob* gene to express itself. Remember that genetics may load the gun, but environment pulls the trigger. If you do have it, you may find it harder to manage your weight with the onset of menstruation, pregnancy, and perimenopause than women who don't have it, and you'll have to work harder to keep it in check.

The bottom line? To paraphrase Frances Kuffel from her autobiographical book, *Passing for Thin*, in which she describes her 170-pound weight-removal journey, "It's not your fault that you have this genetic tendency, but it is your responsibility to do something about it." Pay extra-close attention to your diet and physical activity level as you approach each Milestone.

---

have. The answer, ladies, lies in body composition, which is the body's proportions of muscle, fat, and bone.

All you have to do is look down and around to see that a woman's body composition is dramatically different from a man's. You've got breasts. Hips. A behind. *Thighs.* The average female simply carries more fat and less muscle than the typical male does. For instance, a healthy range of body fat for women up to age 45 is 20 to 25 percent, while a healthy range for men is 10 to 15 percent. Over the age of 45, the range for women extends to approximately 32 percent; men, 25 percent. Furthermore, gender differences in body composition start even before puberty and continue throughout a woman's life. In fact, a baby girl has more fat cells located in her hips, thighs, and buttocks than a baby boy does, who has more fat cells located inside and around his abdomen!

Why the dramatic difference in body fat distribution between men and women? We're still not sure, although differences in hormones, hormone receptors, and concentrations of fat storage enzymes are thought to play a role. But we have learned a thing or two about female fat. For example, research presented at the 2000 annual meeting of the North American Association for the Study of Obesity (NAASO) found that there are not one, not two, but *three* periods in a woman's life when she's most vulnerable to weight gain. The first is at the onset of menstruation, particularly if it arrives early. (Obesity in childhood actually may contribute to early puberty, which in turn increases the risk for more weight gain.) The second is around the time of pregnancy, with a higher risk for women who are already overweight. Finally, many women gain weight between ages 40 and 60, the years during perimenopause and through menopause itself.

Further, recent advances in gender-based medicine have also proven that it's no longer about how fat you are; it's about where that fat ends up. When I started my research work at the NIH, I looked into the question of whether the location of women's body fat might be a predictor for an increased risk of disease. Lo and behold, over the next 10 years, my colleagues and I discovered that excess fat inside the abdomen—which I dubbed Toxic Fat—is lethal, in men and women both. Why "Toxic"? Because too much fat deep inside the abdomen interferes with the liver's ability to manage blood cholesterol and insulin, the hormone that allows your cells to convert food to energy. But we also discovered that, in women, Toxic Fat is associated with an increased risk of heart disease, diabetes, osteoporosis, and cancers of the breast, uterus, and possibly the ovaries. (See, that drive for a flatter stomach is not just about the jeans!)

## YOUR FOUR FEMALE HORMONAL MILESTONES

The National Institutes of Aging (NIA) has funded countless studies that have made it clear that what we thought were the symptoms of aging—increasing girth, mental deterioration, and physical disability—were actually the symptoms of *disuse*. That's why the Body-*for*-LIFE for Women program takes a radically different and more proactive view of female health. If you don't use it, you lose it! And that takes on a different meaning throughout a woman's life. Heck, it's easy to get up and go when you're 15, a mission impossible when you're 8 months pregnant, and a serious time challenge when you're 45. So here are the four female hormonal Milestones, followed by sections devoted to each one, which tell you what you can do to optimize your mental and physical fitness during each.

- Milestone 1: Menstruation to First Pregnancy

- Milestone 2: The Reproductive Years

- Milestone 3: Perimenopause and Menopause

- Milestone 4: Beyond Menopause

Each Milestone represents a significant shift in a woman's hormonal makeup, and each has dramatic implications for her mental and physical health. For example, in Milestone 1, a woman's body is flooded with the female sex hormone estrogen and other female hormones, which help protect her heart and bones, preserve fat stores, and boost mood. In Milestone 4, as estrogen wanes, women need to reframe their approach to physical and emotional well-being.

In each section, I'll talk about how your hormonal Milestones affect your weight, body fat, and overall health. I suggest reading about all the Milestones, as each Milestone is linked to the next. Each will help you understand how your past self-care has influenced your current health, as well as how your current self-care will affect your future well-being. This knowledge can help you see patterns, root out bad habits, and put together a realistic, customized self-care program that will help you achieve your own fittest, healthiest Body-*for*-LIFE.

---

### You Go, Girl! A Milestone 1 Success Story

I work with a lot of overweight teenagers, male and female, and they never fail to inspire me. They work very hard to turn their unhealthy lifestyle habits around, and most succeed. One of my teen patients, a 14-year-old girl named Hilly, is especially inspiring.

"Life was very different 90 pounds ago. At 5 feet 11 inches, 280 pounds, and 50 percent body fat, every day was a struggle. I was tired all the time. I couldn't keep up with my friends. I felt that life was passing me by. I watched a lot of television—reality TV, mostly.

"Thin people don't realize how much harder everything is when you're overweight. Because I spent at least an hour trying on everything in my closet and obsessing over my body in the mirror, I was always at least 20 minutes late for everything. I hated myself. I was sure that everyone was looking at my fat body, making fun of me. As a result, I didn't go out much.

"When I started working with Dr. Peeke, we worked out a plan for me. I was to start taking a brisk walk each day, eat more fruits and veggies, and cut back on the junk food. But she also taught me something equally important: to respect myself, and to show it in how I carried myself. "Fake it until you make it," she said; so I did. I didn't believe just pretending to be confident would work, but it did. Even when I'm feeling insecure, I try to project confidence. It helps me feel a lot stronger.

"It took me a while to get the weight off, but I finally did. I'm 90 pounds lighter, and my body fat is in the healthy high twenties. And I love my daily walk, and I lift my weights. When I get stressed-out, I take a deep breath, get off the couch, put on my sneakers, and go.

"My life is so different now. I get cold in air-conditioned rooms. I love going to the mall and trying on clothes—it's fun, not the nightmare it used to be. And I feel more at home in the world. I realize that obsessing about your body is a waste of time. There are so many other fun things to do—hang out with my friends, go shopping, enjoy the outdoors. I don't watch other people's lives on TV now—I live my own. Now that I'm 90 pounds lighter, reality TV is no match for reality."

## MILESTONE 1: MENSTRUATION TO FIRST PREGNANCY

In this first Milestone, a girl becomes a woman. Essentially, this Milestone encompasses any young woman who hasn't yet been pregnant, so generally speaking, we're talking teens and early twenties here. But even without becoming a mother, a woman in Milestone 1 is on a physical and emotional roller coaster that can be as scary as it is thrilling.

### WHAT'S HAPPENING IN YOUR BODY

Before you hit puberty, your body composition wasn't much different from that of a boy. But when you hit that stage, the surge of estrogen that triggered menstruation also deposited womanly curves on your beanpole body.

This new fat isn't unhealthy fat. This is fat with a mission. It's called essential fat because it's essential to your body's survival—and to your fertility. In men, essential fat (as opposed to excess fat) is about 3 percent of body weight. In women, it runs about 12 percent. Why so much more? Because it includes that gender-specific fat on the hips, thighs, butt, and breasts. Women need it to bear children and to nourish those babies after they're born. Consider this lower body fat to be the body's Exxon station for providing the fuel (calories) needed for breastfeeding. Storage fat, on the other hand, is the fat you accumulate beneath your skin, and includes the deep fat that protects your internal organs. It's also the fat you want to lose—most women carry too much of it.

Your metabolism should be pretty hot in this Milestone. Typically, your physical activity level is higher than it will ever be again, and thus you carry more calorie-burning muscle. Moreover, if you're overweight and decide to remove weight through diet and physical activity, your fat cells are more ready and able to release fat than are those of a woman over 40. Still, excess fat can start to accumulate mighty early.

If you're in Milestone 1, the Body-*for*-LIFE for Women program can help you keep your body composition at its peak. You'll carry a healthy amount of body fat, pack a healthy amount of lean muscle, and have strong, dense bones. If you suffer from premenstrual syndrome (PMS), removing body fat through increased physical fitness and healthy nutrition definitely helps. Add to that better stress management and you can minimize or even eliminate PMS.

## WHAT'S HAPPENING IN YOUR HEAD

This is supposedly the most carefree period of a woman's life. Yeah, right! For many women, this Milestone is the most stressful. Whether in school or slugging it out in the workforce, women in Milestone 1 are pushing the pedal to the metal—they just go and go and go. It's not surprising, then, that they're vulnerable to destructive behaviors of all kinds.

For instance, teenage girls are more likely than boys are to start smoking, and many smoke for stress relief as well as to control their weight. Unfortunately, the consequences of smoking are more serious for females than they are for males. First, females are more likely than men to get hooked on nicotine. Girls who smoke are more likely to have trouble conceiving when they're ready to start a family and more likely to have babies with birth defects. Smoking also raises the risk of osteoporosis. And though it hardly seems fair, a woman who smokes the same amount as a man does is 70 percent more likely to get lung cancer, and at a younger age. Female smokers are also more likely to develop chronic obstructive pulmonary disease (COPD), which causes an unrelenting destruction of the lungs. And smokers can't participate fully in sports when they're gasping for air.

Adolescent girls are also just as likely as boys to experiment with alcohol and binge drinking. It's a biological fact that most women have less of the enzyme that breaks down alcohol. Because of this, they don't metabolize alcohol as efficiently as boys do, so they get drunk faster and stay drunk longer. Drinking can also lead to uninhibited eating and weight gain, especially around the belly. Furthermore, girls who drink are five times more likely to have sex and a third less likely to use condoms.

Because women in Milestone 1 tend to connect their looks with their self-worth, they are particularly vulnerable to eating disorders. In one 1995 study, it was found that 35 percent of "normal" dieters progressed to pathological dieting. Of those, 20 to 25 percent progressed to partial or full-blown eating disorders. Ironically, research suggests that when women regain the weight, as most of them do, they tend to gain it as Toxic Fat, the fat that, in the presence of excess stress hormone, accumulates inside the abdomen. Not only does unchecked stress lead to unhealthy behaviors like smoking, drinking, and disordered eating, but it's also unhealthy in and of itself. In a study from the University of Pittsburgh, researcher Karen Matthews found that young people who didn't adapt well to stress were more likely to go on to develop Toxic Fat, insulin resistance (a first step toward diabetes), and obesity.

## YOUR BIGGEST HEALTH CHALLENGES

All right, it's time for your come-to-heaven lecture. If you're in Milestone 1 and think you can trash your body now and somehow "make up for it" later on, I want a serious attitude adjustment, ladies. How well you take care of yourself now—physically and mentally—determines how well and how long you'll live at 30 and beyond. Here's what you need to pay attention to.

**Clean up your diet.** Get most of your meals at a take-out window? If you want to stay fit and healthy, revamp your eating habits now. One study found that 8 percent of women ages 20 to 34 had severe plaque buildup in their arteries. That plaque is from french fries, doughnuts, sugary cereals, pastries, chips, and late-night pizzas. Though your generous stores of estrogen provide some protection against heart disease now, that shield cracks fast in your forties and fifties, especially if you've abused this vital organ in your youth.

Degreasing and de-sugaring your diet will also protect you from diabetes. Until recently, adult-onset, or type 2, diabetes was most often seen in people over 45. But now an alarming number of young people, including teen girls, are being diagnosed with it. One study of 8,000 men and women found that adults younger than 45 with type 2 diabetes were significantly more likely to have a heart attack than were those who didn't have the condition—and the increased risk was most pronounced in women.

**Establish the exercise habit.** In research by the Heart and Stroke Foundation of Canada, it was found that almost 40 percent of females between ages 12 and 19 were sedentary, as were 53 percent of women in their twenties; U.S. rates are assumed to be similar, if not higher. Even women who were active in high school or college tend to let their exercise habits slide once they hit a workforce filled with high-stress desk jobs, long hours, and lengthy car commutes.

And don't depend upon school anymore to help you with this one. The majority of states no longer require physical education. You have to find something you like to do and practice it regularly. When in doubt, walk more. Join a team. Hang out with active folks. Move!

If you're currently active, fantastic—for heaven's sake, don't change. If you're not, this is your wake-up call. Lace up the sneakers and move it, young ladies. You'll find that even the smallest bit of exercise helps control appetite, burns off harmful stress hormones, improves sleep and mood, and builds self-esteem and confidence—important stuff that most young women have in short supply.

**Protect your bones.** By the time you're 18, you've accumulated 90 percent of the bone mass you'll ever have. After you're 25 or 30, you have to live for the rest of your life on what you've stashed! Chronic dieting, eating disorders, drinking cases of soda, smoking, a low intake of calcium, too much salt, and lack of physical activity all rob valuable bone from the "bank." The result: Women as young as 20 can have the brittle bones of an 80-year-old. Trust me—you don't want to end up in a hospital with a broken hip.

**Treat yourself—and your body—with respect.** So many young women in Milestone 1 hate their bodies. But that loathing isn't an inborn behavior—girls learn to pass judgment on their bodies by comparing them with the "perfect" figures they see in the media. My advice? Bag the skinny media bodies and concentrate on real, fit, and healthy-looking role models. And I mean fit bodies, with curves—go J.Lo, Oprah, and Beyoncé!

Still, the impulse to judge is strong. If you're in Milestone 1, resist judging your body for what it isn't, and optimize what it is—not just to look good but to protect your current and future health. If you love your body and are connected to it rather than disconnected from it, you'll refuse to hurt it with nicotine, alcohol, unprotected sex, and junk food.

**Heads Up!** Build a healthy body composition now. Need a good reason? I'll give you four. First, you'll maintain a hot, calorie-burning metabolism that will sustain you through all four hormonal Milestones. Second, if and when you break an ankle or get sick, your muscle mass hangs in there longer while you heal. Third, lifting weights and eating well give you the curves and glow that turn heads. Finally, eating well and moving your body are the best natural antidepressants a woman can have throughout her life.

## YOUR CUSTOMIZED SOLUTIONS

### Mind

Let's face it, girlfriend: You can't build your career, find a great mate, or even think about having a baby before you get your physical and emotional health together. These tips can help.

**Learn the fine art of stress resilience.** Now is your chance to build your arsenal of de-stressing strategies that will last a lifetime. Body is only as healthy as Mind, and yoga, meditation, or progressive relaxation (among other stress-reduction techniques) can help short-circuit stress overeating (and, by extension, overweight) and help you feel calm, focused, and in control. (You'll find a ton of stress-busting exercises in part 3, Mind: The 10 Body-*for*-LIFE for Women Power Mind Principles.)

**Nip disordered eating now.** If you binge and purge, starve yourself, or exercise compulsively, your body might look great on the outside—but you're headed for trouble. Disordered eating isn't about looking good; it's about sadness, anger, and other funky emotions that are plaguing you. Get help right now—schedule an appointment with a specialist in eating disorders. You can find one in your area by logging on to www.nationaleatingdisorders.org and clicking on "Treatment Referrals."

**Try clubbing with soda.** Social life *is* life for women in Milestone 1. My advice is to have two club sodas for every one alcoholic drink and to choose lower-alcohol drinks, like wine spritzers. You'll have time to metabolize the alcohol you drink, as well as make an intelligent choice as to whether or not you need another. Your liver, your brain, and your body composition (alcohol promotes belly fat) will thank you.

### Mouth

Follow the core Body-*for*-LIFE for Women Eating Method in part 4 as well as these special Milestone 1 tips.

**Don't skip meals, especially the first one.** I still meet countless women who skip meals, particularly breakfast, to remove weight. They're not doing themselves any favors. A study by the U.S. National Weight Control Registry of 3,000 men and women found that of those who successfully maintained weight loss, nearly 80 percent ate breakfast regularly. Fueling in the morning provides valuable appetite control later in the day and is a great predictor for sustained success in staying fit.

**Scale back the happy-hour habit.** Alcohol + high-fat foods (like buffalo wings) = excess body fat. Studies show that people who simultaneously indulge in the two burn fewer calories and store more fat, so limit your brews and avoid those fatty favorites.

**Drink smarter beverages.** Americans drink 14 billion gallons of soda each year—that's 54 gallons for every man, woman, and child. This liquid candy is bad for your bones, weight, and blood sugar. Instead, keep a bottle of water around at all times, opt for an icy-cold glass of seltzer with a squeeze of lemon, or try one of those flavored sports waters sweetened with sucralose (they're about 10 calories a bottle). Even better, keep building those bones with three 8-ounce glasses of skim milk each day. Science has even shown that the calcium in milk can make your fat cells more efficient at weight removal.

**Experiment with new ways of eating.** The largest group of new vegetarians in this country are men and women under the age of 25. Some are "fish vegetarians," and others don't eat fish, eggs, or dairy. Some just cut out red meat, and others choose ethnic variations. This is also a grand opportunity to learn how to cook, since it really requires you to work with whole foods. If you're interested in experimenting with vegetarianism, there are a slew of great cookbooks that can get you started.

**Mind your nutrients.** Take one multivitamin every morning. This will also remind you to have breakfast. Although you should be getting all of your vitamins and minerals from whole foods, you know as well as I do that you're not eating anywhere near the five to nine servings of fruit and veggies you should be getting.

## Muscle

For your best body, follow the core Body-*for*-LIFE for Women Training Method in part 5 as well as these special Milestone 1 tips.

**Move your body.** One of the easiest ways to maintain a healthy weight is simply to be more active in your everyday life. Walk to school. Bike to work. Park in one spot downtown and walk to all the shops you need to get to, rather than driving to each of them separately. Every extra step brings you closer to achieving your Body-*for*-LIFE.

**Get a life!** Some surveys show that the average television viewing time per day, per home is 6 hours, 47 minutes. If everyone watched just *half* that much, we'd be a thinner, healthier nation! Vow to cut TV time in half, and you'll have almost 25 hours a week to fill with active, interesting living.

## MILESTONE 2: THE REPRODUCTIVE YEARS

Most likely, your life is more settled than it was in Milestone 1. You might be married, with children, perhaps well-established in your career. Or maybe you're a stay-at-home mom or you're reentering the workforce. Whatever you're doing, I know you're up to your eyeballs in life. For just a moment, visualize a typical day. Do you spend more time at work and less at the gym? Drive when you used to walk? Take the elevator instead of bounding up the stairs? Go to the movies more and go dancing less? Are you stressed-out and heading for the vending machine at work or the fridge at night for comfort? If so, you may find the number on your scale edging north, and a few days of careful eating won't get rid of those extra pounds as quickly as they once did. No wonder the average woman gains a minimum of 20 pounds between ages 20 and 65.

Welcome to Milestone 2.

### WHAT'S HAPPENING IN YOUR BODY

Starting at around age 25 or 30, a woman's basal metabolic rate—the rate at which she burns calories at rest—can begin to decline, if she's less physically active and starts losing precious muscle. A pound of muscle needs about 35 to 50 calories per day to function; a pound of fat, fewer than 3 calories. It's simple: The less muscle you have, the fewer calories you'll burn.

If you're pregnant or planning to be, you'll have better luck removing those post-pregnancy pounds if you eat well and are physically active before you conceive. If you're already overweight, the hormonal mayhem of pregnancy may make it a challenge to remove those pounds. (But don't throw up your hands just yet—you *can* get your body back.) Basically, the second that fertilized egg hits your uterus, it triggers a hormonal avalanche. During pregnancy, special enzymes called lipoprotein lipase (LPL) charge into high gear in the butt, hip, and thigh region. These enzymes promote fat storage in both fat and muscle cells. This sets up a kind of baby "feeding station" in your lower body so that you'll have plenty of fuel to draw on once you've delivered and start breastfeeding.

But pregnancy does not automatically doom a woman to permanent overweight. The most crucial factor is the *pattern* of your weight gain. What you want to do is gain slowly and steadily in the first and second trimesters, and put on most of your weight in the third trimester, when your baby is growing the fastest. In one study of pregnant women, excess weight gain early on was a significant factor in how much weight they retained after they gave birth.

Whether or not you've had children, the good news is that women in Milestone 2 can maintain their strength and their lean body mass—even improve them, if need be. Although cardio (walking, jogging, cycling) is crucial for a woman's health and well-being, it's resistance training that will make the biggest impact on her not-as-young-as-it-used-to-be body. Here's a crucial Body-*for*-LIFE for Women rule: For every decade of a woman's life starting with age 20, resistance training becomes more and more important to her survival. It keeps her muscles, bones, and mind strong, and as you'll learn in part 5, resistance training revs up your metabolic rate so you burn more calories, even at rest. So fret not—you can still be fit, firm, and sexy while you safeguard your future health. Following the Body-*for*-LIFE for Women Eating and Training Methods in this book will show you how.

## WHAT'S HAPPENING IN YOUR HEAD

Men come home from work and relax. Women? Ha! None of that "Honey, I'm home" stuff for you. At 5:00 P.M. you leave the office—if you're lucky—and come home to start your second shift.

In most cases, women in Milestone 2 still bear primary responsibility for getting dinner on the table, doing household chores, and making time for their children. Many of them are now the primary providers of the family income. Keeping all those balls in the air is stressful. I don't have to tell you that, I know. But have you really ever stopped to think about just how stressful?

Well, think about it now. There's no break—no period of transition between the demands of work and the equally challenging demands of home life. The pressure many women experience in trying to be all things to all people—and trying to get it all done, and done well—can be just as taxing as a major stressor like death, illness, or divorce. If, each and every week, you're carting Johnny to karate class and Janie to soccer, and keeping it together at work and at home without going postal, you are a hero, honey. But even Superwoman didn't spend all her time in her breastplate and cape. If you routinely function under a lot of stress, even one tiny extra stressor can send you over the edge.

Somehow women always seem to survive the crisis. But often it's at the expense of their own physical and mental health. Most women in this Milestone seek relief from stress by overeating. Others smoke, or abuse drugs and alcohol. Women in Milestone 2 tend to take their comfort where they can get it. But the trick is to neutralize stresses in healthy, life-affirming ways, rather than self-destructive ones. I'll give you a hint: A huge part of shedding that crushing load of worry and stress comes from making the time—no, assertively *taking* the time—to eat the way you know you should, and to sweat out stress in yoga class, on a walk, or with the weights. You'll find out how in the next few parts of this book.

## YOUR BIGGEST HEALTH CHALLENGES

From making child-care decisions to riding the hormonal highs and lows of PMS or pregnancy, this Milestone can deliver unprecedented levels of stress. Your main challenge is to just keep yourself on your daily radar and seek a balance—some time for yourself and some time for all the rest. You can honor your commitment to yourself as well as your family. Here are your marching orders.

**Maintain a healthy weight.** Your basic nutrition needs don't change much between Milestones 1 and 2, but your calorie needs do. Face it: If you're not as active as you once were, you just don't need as much food as you used to. If you don't make the time to burn off your daily calories, then you have to cut back. Otherwise, you'll wear 'em! Consume an extra 250 calories per day, and you'll be 25 pounds heavier by this time next year. I'd rather just get more active and continue to eat well. A nice win-win.

**Care for the caregiver.** That's you. As I've mentioned, women are caregivers supreme, and the better they tend to those they love, the more they neglect their own care and maintenance. You have to be your own caregiver and give yourself your own love and support. That means joining the health club and actually showing up. Self-care takes focus, dedication, and planning. It also takes a major shift in thinking: You've got to come to believe that your health and happiness are just as important as your family's.

**Make time for physical activity.** Moving your body is not a burden. It's a gift to yourself—what I call "a pocket of peace"—in which you regroup and refuel so that you can fully embrace and enjoy life. Exercise relieves pent-up energy and muscle tension and strengthens your heart, which bears the brunt of the physiological stress response. It also improves self-esteem. While a 10-minute walk can defuse a stressful situation, regular exercise can help stamp out stress before it starts. The Body-*for*-LIFE for Women Training Method can help your body—and mind—rise to the challenges of everyday life.

**Heads Up!** You may be years away from menopause, but if you're carrying extra weight, remove it now. If you don't, chances are that the excess poundage will hang on into your postmenopausal years. If you're now pregnant or planning a pregnancy, limit your pregnancy weight gain to between 25 and 35 pounds. A study conducted at Georgetown University found that women who gained more than 40 pounds during pregnancy faced a 40 percent greater risk of developing breast cancer after menopause. Women who retained the added pounds after their pregnancies were at the greatest risk, regardless of their starting weight.

## YOUR CUSTOMIZED SOLUTIONS

In Milestone 2, your mission is to learn to make time to take care of yourself. Yes, you have to learn, and I've taught untold numbers of women how to do it. Follow these tips to help yourself meet the unique challenges of this busy Milestone while still getting in that all-important self-care.

### Mind

Once you hit this Milestone, you need more than a tub of bubbles to ease the stress you face each day. Recognize that balancing your life is as important as balancing your checkbook.

**Learn to prioritize.** Most women have a chronic case of "helium hand." When asked to do anything (take on one more work project, agree to schlep carloads of kids to events, bake cookies for the PTA meeting), their hands drift upward, and before they can say "Did I do that?" they've gone and signed up for one more thing.

Look, no one can cram 25 hours' worth of life into 24. A smarter solution is to learn to cut through the unnecessary "filler" in your day—the stuff you *think* you have to do but really don't.

Don't believe anything in your schedule is expendable? Write out a typical day's to-do list. Include everything—board meetings, your PTA or volunteer obligations, walking the dog, banking, picking up the dry cleaning. After you complete your list, ask yourself:

- Is this a must-do activity or task?

- Is it important to me?

- Can I delegate it?

- Can I trash it?

- Does it interfere with my self-care?

Don't start pondering about how people might think about this or that. Just focus, and seek ways to find the time it will take to add some self-care balance into your life. Once you actually sit down and think about your obligations, you'll be surprised at how many you can delegate to someone else (your husband, perhaps?) or simply jettison.

**Learn a healthy response to stress.** Research by Herbert Benson, M.D., and Jon Kabat-Zinn, Ph.D., showed that if a woman learns to elicit a state of deep physical rest on command, her body and mind return to a calm, relaxed state. Heart rate, blood pressure, stress hormone levels, and muscle tension drop. This state of deep calm is called the relaxation response, and it's incredibly simple to do. Practice this technique once or twice daily.

**Step 1.** Pick a focus word or short phrase.

**Step 2.** Sit quietly in a comfortable position and close your eyes.

**Step 3.** Relax your muscles. Breathe slowly and naturally, and as you do, repeat your focus word, phrase, or prayer silently to yourself as you exhale.

**Step 4.** Don't worry about how well you're doing. When other thoughts come to mind, say to yourself, "Oh, well," and gently return to the repetition. Continue for 10 to 20 minutes.

**Step 5.** Do not stand immediately. Continue sitting quietly for a minute or so. Then open your eyes and sit for another minute before rising.

**Make quality sleep a priority.** To women in Milestone 2, sleep is a precious and often elusive gift, and in my experience, sleep-deprived women are more apt to mindlessly overeat. Women often eat to maintain energy, when what they really need is longer nighttime sleep or a daytime nap. So fight for your right to refreshing, uninterrupted shut-eye. Get to bed and turn that TV off no later than 11:00 P.M. (ideally, 10:00 P.M.). Tape a late-night show you want to see, and watch it the next day while you're working out on the treadmill or the elliptical trainer. Use soothing music, a bath, a book, meditation—anything to help you unwind.

## Mouth

You're probably the one who gets dinner on the table. Planning for these meals is a great opportunity to assess the quality and quantity of healthy foods in your diet. Follow the core Body-*for*-LIFE for Women Eating Method in part 4 as well as these special Milestone 2 tips.

**Get enough protein.** You'll learn all about your protein needs in the next part of this book, but aim to get 20 to 30 percent of your daily calories from protein-rich sources like fish, poultry, lean red meat, beans, soy products, and low-fat dairy. Protein promotes satiety, or a feeling of fullness. It helps you build precious calorie-burning muscle. Besides, the body uses 20 to 30 percent more energy to digest protein than it does to digest carbs or fat.

**Watch the late-night eating.** If you overeat at any time of the day, you will gain weight. The evening hours are especially precarious because you probably won't use all those calories you consume; you'll store some or most of them as fat. Also, you're likely to be tired, so you won't pay attention to serving size, and stressed-out, so you'll seek comfort in eating. Try to finish dinner before 8 o'clock at least 4 to 5 days per week. Brush your teeth, and stay away from the kitchen. In part 4, you'll find out more about how and when to eat.

**Mind your nutrients.** If you're 40 or under, pregnant or not, and generally healthy, take a multivitamin every day. If you're like most women, you're not getting all the servings of fruits and veggies you need to maintain an adequate amount of antioxidants, vitamins, and minerals to support your health. Think of your multi as a little extra "health insurance."

## Muscle

Heart-pounding, lung-filling exercise—both cardio and resistance training—burns calories and elevates metabolism. To start reaping the physical and mental benefits of regular exercise, follow the core Body-*for*-LIFE for Women Training Method in part 5 as well as these special Milestone 2 tips.

**Step it up!** Did you get a pedometer yet? Well, run out and get one right now! It can be a busy Milestone 2 woman's best friend. Inexpensive and low-tech, it doesn't require any expertise, and just wearing it will remind you to add more movement to your everyday life. To start, wear a pedometer for at least 3 days—from the time you get out of bed until you go to sleep at night—to determine how much activity you're currently getting. Try to measure at least 1 weekend day, because activity levels will vary from weekdays. Add 500 to 1,000 steps a day until you reach your daily goal of 10,000 steps per day. (You'll find a pedometer plan in part 5.)

**Take the pain out of cardio.** Milestone 2 women get so little downtime that I think it's fine to watch a video or TV while you do your aerobic exercise—as long as you sweat, which is a measure of how hard you're working. If you have a treadmill, an elliptical trainer, or a stepper at home, put a small TV—which has a remote—near the equipment. Music channels can be particularly fun to work out to. Tune in your Walkman, or load some music into your MP3 player, and take it with you wherever you walk, run, bike, or work out. There's nothing like great tunes when you want to pump it up.

**Participate in a sports event.** If stress and fatigue have put a damper on your motivation, consider signing up for a walk, bike ride, or run to raise public awareness of a health issue important to women, like breast cancer or diabetes. Not only will you stay focused on your training, but you'll feel like you've done something worthwhile—that has meaning for you. Which, when you're in the eye of the hurricane that is Milestone 2, is a very big deal.

## MILESTONE 3: PERIMENOPAUSE AND MENOPAUSE

Welcome to Milestone 3! This is where I'm hanging out right now, and I'm happy to tell you that the view from here is just fine. You might think I'm crazy. What's so

---

**Teach Your Daughter a Thing or Two about Health**

If you're in Milestone 3 and have a daughter in Milestone 1, now is the time to get her involved in healthy eating and exercise habits.

Mothers greatly underestimate how much influence they have over their daughters' health habits. Fact is, if you have a daughter, she's been watching you for years and taking copious mental notes. If you tell her to eat her broccoli but don't touch the stuff yourself, she learns that adults don't take their own advice. Likewise for exercise. Don't think you can just open the front door and say, "Go play." She's not a baby anymore; she's becoming a woman, and she needs to learn from you how to be a healthy one.

One of my patients, Lisa, is an awesome role model to her daughter. She's an active woman and has always encouraged her daughter, 13-year-old Cassie, to come along on her walks, runs, hikes, and bike rides. At an age when many of her peers were worried about their weight, Cassie was strong and self-assured. She played soccer and lacrosse and was proud of her muscles.

It's important to note that Lisa wasn't the food police, either. She kept cookies and candy in the house, and she and her daughter ate their share of pizza and fast food. But overall, their meals were healthy and balanced. Cassie learned that there was room in her diet for occasional goodies, as long as she stayed active and ate well most of the time.

Cassie is now 17 and in fabulous shape. So is her mom, now 45 and a fit, strong 5 feet 5 inches, with a body fat of 19 percent, and 135 pounds. Though Lisa and Cassie developed their healthy habits early in life, it's important that moms realize that it's never, ever too late to influence their daughters' health.

---

cool about more body fat, a wider waist, and a metabolism that appears to be tanking? The good news is that you can get control of all this, and look and feel better than you ever have.

Typically in Milestone 3, your kids, if you have any, are older; your time is more your own. Your stresses may include workplace woes, the boomerang child who's back in his or her old room until that elusive job appears, or new worries about age-related medical conditions of you or your loved ones. For the first time in your life, you're thinking about your own mortality. I'll never forget my first conversations with my good friend Katie Couric, who, while in her early forties, suffered through the tragic loss of both her young husband and her older sister. It's such a cruel blow to have to endure that grief and look into the mirror of your own life and worry about death.

And then there's the other big M—menopause. But first you have to get through perimenopause, which, as currently defined by the NIH, extends from the first onset of symptoms through the 12 months after the cessation of your menses. This phase can extend from the late thirties to the midfifties. Ouch. That's a lot of time to be shape-shifting in your hormonal hurricane, soaking in your bedsheets, waking up all night, hot-flashing, and enduring funky, unpredictable menstrual cycles.

I know through experience that you're really frustrated about midlife weight gain. Well, we'll get it off you, girlfriend. But let me tell you this: In this Milestone, it's definitely about removing fat and looking great while living through a natural estrogen withdrawal. But it's also about optimizing every opportunity for perimenopausal self-care now, so that you can continue to live well in the future.

## WHAT'S HAPPENING IN YOUR BODY

After age 40, the average woman starts losing about $\frac{1}{2}$ pound of muscle per year. Actually, through disuse, she can lose 5 to 10 pounds of muscle between ages 40 and 55. As I've already mentioned, when you lose muscle, your daily calorie burn dips, while the number of calories you eat either stays the same or increases. Either way, you end up with more body fat. Now, add that to declining female sex hormones, a sedentary lifestyle, and the presence of what I call "Toxic Stress," and you have the recipe for big-time weight gain during this period of life.

Where's the fat going? If you're 40 or over, you know. The upper body gets fluffier.

Estrogen usually directs fat to the lower body, but as hormone levels begin to decline, it becomes easier to deposit extra fat on the upper body. You get the back roll, the flapping upper arms, the fat that pooches out over your bra (one of my patients refers to it as having two extra breasts). Speaking of bras, don't be surprised if you go up at least a cup size.

And you get the single most frustrating symptom of this Milestone—the expanding waistline. Suddenly *belt* is a four-letter word. Like men, women in Milestone 3 store excess belly fat in two compartments. The first is outside the abdominal muscle. I call it the "menopot" (manopot, for men!). The second is underneath the abdominal wall, around the organs, deep in the belly. Yep, Toxic Fat.

Some studies have found that postmenopausal women have up to 49 percent more intra-abdominal fat and 36 percent more upper-body fat than premenopausal women do. The grand majority of women will get a menopot. It's normal and to be expected as you course through perimenopause. Typically, the menopot is no more than about 5 pounds and is not associated with illness. We'll always have some menopot as we age. The key is to minimize it to its rock bottom and keep it like that.

But it isn't as easy as when we were premenopausal. Menopot fat is stubborn fat. Studies conducted at the University of Maryland showed that these Milestone 3 fat cells are less efficient at releasing their fat to be used as energy. This means that the menopot is probably a throwback to prehistoric times, when the matriarch of the clan needed extra body fat to survive famine so she could care for her children and grandchildren.

This shift of fat from our behinds to the menopot saved our female butts back in prehistoric times. But it's the Toxic Fat we should really be worried about.

If excess fat starts to accumulate inside your abdomen, you've got problems. As I noted, Toxic Fat raises a woman's risk for heart disease, diabetes, and cancer. What's more, as you lose estrogen and gain body fat, your levels of protective HDL cholesterol drop, while your levels of artery-clogging LDL cholesterol and triglycerides rise.

Though growing a small menopot is inevitable—I have mine!—a full-blown gut is not. So don't expect to completely eliminate your menopot. Just minimize it with good nutrition and regular physical activity. When researchers at the University of

Pittsburgh Medical Center compared the body compositions of athletic peri-menopausal women with those of women who were couch potatoes or who were only moderately active, they found that the athletes had the least trunk, arm, leg, and total body fat. Plus, they weighed an average of 17 pounds less than the less active gals.

## WHAT'S HAPPENING IN YOUR HEAD

Just when you get adept at making time for yourself, managing stress and your career, and organizing a household while caring for everyone and his brother, wham! Your mind and body mutiny on you. Welcome to perimenopause.

If you had wild mood swings during pregnancy or each month before your period, you may find that they come flooding back. You may get weepy, and then let loose with the telephone operator. Blame that on the ebb and flow of your sex hormones, which have a profound effect on mood.

Add to this more or increasing stresses in your life. Of all the Milestones, Milestone 3 is characterized by the most complex, and often the greatest amount of, caregiving in your life. You may have preteen or teen children and an aging mother to contend with, along with your partner, a job—the whole "catastrophe" as author Jon Kabat-Zinn would say—so you're pulled at both ends to provide endless hours of selfless service. This tends to worsen any symptoms of aging and perimenopause you may already be experiencing.

Women tell me they find that their brains seem to be short-circuiting. They'll be speaking in a meeting or to a friend on the phone, and suddenly they can't think of the word or number they want to use. They may go into the bedroom or the supermarket and forget what they went in for. You know—the lost-keys-and-glasses syndrome. The fuzzies. I hear that a lot from my patients in Milestone 3. Your energy may tank, too. Getting out of bed is a challenge; you crumple by 3:00 P.M. and collapse when you get home. And then begin the strange events. At work, you are horrified to find that one of your shoes is navy and the other is black. (I've done this twice. Thank God, they were dark colors.) Or you look in the mirror and find that you've put on only one earring—the other is on your vanity table at home.

Like the mood swings of this Milestone, the fuzzies are thought to be caused by fluctuating levels of estrogen. You accept that they're a normal piece of this perimenopausal process, and you learn to plan around it. Me? I always carry a notepad and tons of Post-its.

Bottom line, most women feel like they're losing their minds. Nope! You're going through estrogen withdrawal, and your body needs some time to adjust while you're helping it along with a healthy lifestyle. I can assure you that the confusion and memory loss is almost always fleeting and completely normal. When you care for your body with physical exercise, your mind benefits, too. The more blood and oxygen circulating up there, the better your brain will function.

## YOUR BIGGEST HEALTH CHALLENGES

Each woman's perimenopause is different—different physical signs, different emotional responses. That said, here are the most common physical and mental challenges you may face.

**Avoid Toxic Stress.** Well, you can't completely avoid it, but you sure can minimize it. Stress adds one more hormone to the menopausal boiling pot—the stress hormone cortisol. As you'll learn in part 4 of this book, chronic elevation of cortisol encourages the body to store fat intra-abdominally. Making matters worse, many women turn to food for comfort during times of stress. And it ain't exactly tuna on a bed of greens.

Here's the deal. Women are already at high risk for stress-eating of carbs and fats. Add to that mix unpredictable, fluctuating sex hormones that influence appetite—coupled with new evidence that women's ability to sense sweet taste is impaired, making them seek sweeter foods in general—and you have the perfect conditions for piling on boatloads of Toxic Fat. As women discover that their traditional Milestone 1 and 2 weight-loss techniques no longer work, they get more stressed-out, which results in more eating and the storage of even more Toxic Fat. If this cycle remains unchecked, you're looking at an increased risk of heart disease, diabetes, and cancer, not to mention escalating depression and anxiety. All the more reason to check out the stress-reduction techniques in part 3.

**Manage perimenopausal symptoms.** You may not have them at all. But evidence suggests that one-third to one-half of women at midlife experience symptoms associated with perimenopause, including hot flashes, night sweats, insomnia, fatigue, mood swings, and memory changes. However, research shows that midlife women who manage their hormones with lifestyle changes—diet, exercise, stress-control strategies—have fewer problems with menopausal symptoms than do those who stay stuck in their sedentary, stressed-out, junk-food-laden ways.

**Heads Up!** Most women will spend one-third to one-half of their lifetimes in Milestone 4. So you need a game plan. Do you want to paint? Cook? Travel the world? Start a whole new career? Dare to dream—and then start putting the plans into place to make it happen.

Whatever your plans, make sure they include physical fitness. In the Women's Health Initiative, a study of more than 160,000 postmenopausal women ages 50 to 79, researchers found that the longer a woman sat each day, the greater her risk of cardiovascular disease, even after they adjusted for time spent in recreational activity.

And in keeping with our Mind-Mouth-Muscle theme, the perimenopausal years are when you have to pay attention to your *mental* aerobics as well as your physical activity. Harvard University researchers have found that a common characteristic of centenarians is that they continually challenge their brains, which has helped them maintain amazing mental clarity and memory. So remember, for *all* of your muscles—physical and mental—if and you don't use 'em, you lose 'em!

## YOUR CUSTOMIZED SOLUTIONS

Your body is in transition; your emotions may be, too. Taking good care of yourself now, through a healthy diet and regular exercise, can help you feel more in control of this turbulent time of life. Follow the program in parts 3, 4, and 5; plus, take addition steps to address the issues that emerge in this Milestone.

## Mind

You're undergoing a profound transition on every level—physical, mental, emotional, spiritual. Yet you're still all things to all people—parent, partner, caregiver to aging parents, career woman. It's a tall order, but you can navigate this Milestone without losing your mind. Here's how.

**Fight the fuzzies.** Because you can't afford to be derailed at home or at work by a sometimes-sputtering brain, start investigating the wonderful world of organizing and reminder tools. Stick Post-it notes onto your computer at work or onto your bathroom mirror. Invest in a handheld computer—I couldn't survive without mine— or simply carry a small notebook in which you've written your to-do list, and refer to it frequently.

<u>Create a sense of calm.</u> The quality of your living and working environment is critical to maintaining mental peace, not to mention sanity. The atmosphere in which you live can relieve stress or create it. How about muted lighting and pastel colors? Or aromatherapy? Also, research shows that music physically alters your brain waves, either exciting or calming them. Take a trip to your local CD store and check out soothing tunes. I have the music of flutist Debbie Danbrook of Healing Music playing softly in the background at my office. It makes a big difference for me as well as my stressed-out patients.

**Recruit a helping hand.** Just because you're part of the sandwich generation (taking care of your kids as well as older parents) doesn't mean you have to be per- petually squeezed. You simply can't do it all. Once a week, set yourself free for an afternoon. Give yourself permission to step back and let someone else take the care- giving reins for a while. Ask your partner or a sibling to help out. Find an adult day care for an elderly parent, or swap kid-watching with a neighbor. Be assertive about asking for help and support. More often than not, if you don't ask, you won't get.

## Mouth

For years, you might have eaten whatever you wanted and kind of gotten away with it. Well, after the age of 40, the party's over. Even if you're doing great with phys- ical activity, terrific. But you still have to pay close attention to your daily calories. To optimize the healthy eating required for this Milestone, follow the Body-*for*-LIFE for Women eating advice in part 4, along with these special tips for Milestone 3.

<u>Eat less—and better.</u> During Milestone 3, you might be eating out more often because of professional work or because you're just not cooking as much anymore. In light of this situation, you need to pay more attention to servings and portion sizes—even if you're eating most meals at home. Don't resent the extra effort. In- stead, realize that you'll enjoy higher-quality food while cutting the quantity a bit. Think of it this way. Do you want a pile of zircons, or one incredible diamond? Ten

cruddy cookies, or one mouthwatering one? Go for the diamond, and you'll look like one.

**Scratch the sugar.** As I mentioned, women in Milestone 3 are especially attracted to sugary foods. Research now shows that many women over the age of 40 experience a heightened interest in sweets because of a dampening of their perception of sweet taste. That means we're actually craving more sweetness to get the same level of sweet taste we had before. Be careful here, and learn how to sweeten foods without eating a mountain of sugar. Use applesauce, the herb stevia, sucralose, and citrus juices as satisfying alternatives. Also, the longer you go without eating foods made with white sugar, the less you'll crave them.

**Spare the starches.** The high-quality starches are the multigrain breads and pastas, brown rice, and sweet potatoes. Although these are healthful foods, they usually don't come in single-serving packages. It's hard for a stressed-out, distracted woman to pay attention to how much she's serving herself, especially at night, when's she's weary and foggy-headed. So my advice is to eat two or three servings of high-quality starches during the day. Then, 5 nights a week, just eliminate them from your dinner plate. Save one or two servings of these high-quality starches for a Friday night out at your favorite restaurant, or Sunday dinner with the family.

What about white rice, white bread, and refined pasta? Lose 'em. They're guaranteed to set off a rip-roaring appetite for more of this junk.

**Eat woman food.** You're not a man. Why eat like one? Especially when in the presence of men, remember that you need "woman food" and woman-size portions. At business lunches or dinners or at family gatherings, don't mindlessly eat exactly what some 6-foot-3 hairy-chested guy is inhaling. Also, when you're out and about, you know that serving sizes at restaurants and fast-food joints are completely out of control; a plate of pasta may contain seven or eight servings, and a sandwich is big enough to serve a Super Bowl party. This national super-sizing has trickled down to our own home cooking. Cut your portions in half (except for nonstarchy veggies—pile those on!), and have four or five servings of fruit each day. Pay attention, be mindful, and try to eat more slowly—consciously put down your fork 10 times throughout your meal. When you're done, sip your drink and let your food sit for 5 minutes before you decide if you're still hungry. If you are, eat a second serving, but take only half of what you'd usually take. Most of my patients are surprised by how little food is required to fill them up.

**Rack up the calcium.** Milestone 3 is your last call for calcium. Most North American women eat a pitiful 600 milligrams a day—that's only about half the amount they need for healthy bones. Include a calcium-rich food like milk, yogurt, or dark green leafy vegetables at every meal, and if you drink orange juice, buy the calcium-fortified kind.

**Minimize red meat.** Many cancer experts advise women to consume no more than 3 ounces of red meat a day, period, because they believe there's a link between high meat consumption and breast cancer. Makes sense to me, especially considering that in countries where meat is used almost as a condiment—merely to add a little flavor to food—there are significantly lower rates of breast cancer than in the United States. For protein, I recommend an emphasis on heart-healthy fish, poultry, or vegetarian combinations.

**Give soy a chance.** Soybeans contain plant estrogens called isoflavones, compounds that have a weak estrogen-like effect in the body. Long-term studies show that perimenopausal and menopausal women who eat a diet rich in whole-food plant estrogens—tofu or edamame (whole soybeans)—have fewer hot flashes and less vaginal dryness, and maintain greater bone density, than those who eat few plant estrogens. Other studies suggest that an isoflavone-rich diet may prevent heart disease, improve cholesterol, and help prevent breast cancer.

It's easier than ever to eat soy these days. You can buy soy protein burgers, hot dogs, ground "beef," deli "meats," and more. Make sure to buy products made from the whole bean and not from extractions. (The label will usually say "made from whole soybeans.") Or simply pour yourself a glass of low-fat soy milk. In a study from the Bowman Gray School of Medicine in North Carolina, researchers found that women who drink just 8 ounces of soy milk a day have fewer hot flashes than do women who drink a similar nonsoy beverage.

**Limit alcohol.** Don't have more than one alcoholic drink a day—maybe a small glass of wine with dinner. I'm a fan of the wine spritzer—half a glass of white wine and the rest sparkling water. Nurse it and savor the flavor. Although studies suggest that moderate drinking can help protect a woman's heart and reduce her risk of diabetes and maybe even Alzheimer's disease, alcohol is also calorie dense. One glass of wine or beer contains about 100 calories. If you prefer mixed drinks, like margaritas, you're drinking even more calories. And I don't think I have to tell you that when you have a few drinks in your system, your good judgment goes out the window and you're more likely to overeat. You probably found that out in Milestone 1!

**Mind your nutrients.** In addition to your daily multi, take:

- 1,000 milligrams of omega-3 fatty acids (2,000 milligrams a day if you have early signs of heart disease, and up to 4,000 milligrams a day if you have had a heart attack or stroke)

- 1,200 to 1,500 milligrams of calcium

- 100 milligrams of coenzyme $Q_{10}$ to prevent heart disease and some mental conditions, such as Parkinson's disease

- One baby aspirin to prevent heart disease and breast cancer

## Muscle

Studies have shown that women who ramp up their physical activity during this Milestone gain far less weight than do those who decrease their activity. Other studies have shown a fairly direct connection between the decrease in physical activity and both the decrease in resting metabolic rate and the increase in fat mass during menopause. Follow the core Body-*for*-LIFE for Women Training Method in part 5 as well as these special Milestone 3 tips.

**Minimize your menopot.** If your menopot has gotten out of control, parts 4 and 5 of this book will help you shrink it. Red alert: The longer you let it go, the harder it is to get it under control. So hop to it.

**Battle batwings.** Unless you've been working out with weights all along, the backs of your arms—the triceps region—may be heading south, giving you those dreaded flapping batwings you remember your grade school teachers having. The Body-*for*-LIFE for Women Training Method exercises, shown in Appendix A, will help stave them off. The ones to focus on: triceps kickbacks.

**Always warm up properly.** As you age, flexibility is key to maintaining optimal mobility and preventing bone fractures should you slip and fall. After age

40, your joints, ligaments, and muscles might not be as flexible and elastic as they used to be, so whether you're doing cardio or resistance training, be sure to incorporate a 5- to 10-minute warmup period into your training regimen. Several minutes of walking, followed by gentle stretches, will help prevent you from getting hurt or overly sore.

**Cultivate a sense of adventure.** Seize the day, and use each event as a valuable lesson and an opportunity to experiment and grow, mind and body. Don't be afraid to get out there and make new friends and enjoy new adventures. Women who have active hobbies are more likely to continue exercising for their whole lives than are those who simply follow a mindless exercise "routine." That's because they consider their activity playtime rather than an obligatory workout. Now's a great time to start investigating new activities. Because your kids are probably a little older, they can take care of themselves more, and you may also have a healthy amount of vacation time stored up to pursue a fun new activity. Pick up some adventure magazines and see what speaks to you. You don't have to be an athlete to take up invigorating but easy-to-learn sports like sea kayaking, mountain hiking, bicycling, or snowshoeing. Women who keep mentally and physically active look and feel like it as well.

Not really into the great outdoors? There's plenty to do indoors as well. Join clubs, be a community volunteer, take up art classes, go back to school. Try Pilates, explore the martial arts, or sign up for a dance class at your local Y. The more you try, the more likely you'll find something you love to do for life.

## MILESTONE 4: BEYOND MENOPAUSE

Most women notice the first round of physical changes around age 50, and then again sometime around the 7th decade. (Hey—if you've been rocking and rolling on this planet for nearly 70 years, expect to have a few creaking joints to show for it.) You'll have a few more aches and pains, and your body composition will start to change as you lose a little more muscle mass and, relatively speaking, increase your percentage of body fat.

Don't panic. In part 5, you'll learn that body fat percentage is total pounds of body

## Esther—70 and Still Going Strong

When Esther came to see me several years ago, she was in despair. Her husband of 40 years had recently died. The arthritis in her knees made it difficult for her to walk, let alone exercise. Her 36-inch waist was expanding, her body fat was 37 percent, and her cholesterol and blood pressure were on the rise. The only thing dropping were Esther's spirits as she fell into a deeper and deeper funk.

In the course of our conversations, Esther revealed how lonely she'd been since her husband died. She'd been stress-overeating at night to compensate for his absence. I encouraged her to accept invitations to social gatherings, which she did. Before long, she was making new friends, both male and female.

I also told Esther to cut out refined sugars and white starches and limit her consumption of healthy starches, like sweet potatoes and brown rice, to smaller portions early in the day. She dropped the after-dinner eating and replaced it with phone calls and gatherings with friends.

Because walking was hard, Esther joined water aerobics, which got her heart pumping but was gentle on her sore joints. She also began lifting weights in a special senior class, where the instructors knew how to work around everyday aches. It was a win-win, because she also made friends and picked up new activities to do with them each week.

Over the course of 6 months, Esther's waistline shrank 4 inches, and she bubbled over with energy and optimism. Her blood pressure and cholesterol levels normalized. She still had knee pain, but her flexibility, strength, and endurance improved. And now she has the energy to keep up with her grandchildren.

fat divided by total weight (which is total pounds of fat, muscle, bones, organs, and water). This means that even if your body fat stays the same, if you lose muscle mass, your percentage of fat increases. So fear not. These numbers are totally normal, totally natural. Just as a 45-year-old woman shouldn't expect to have the abs of a 20-year-old, a 60-year-old woman needs to understand that she'll be a little softer. But that doesn't mean cream-filled-doughnut soft. The key is to stay off that rocker and keep on rolling.

## WHAT'S HAPPENING IN YOUR BODY

Until recently, it was assumed that getting shrunken and frail was a natural part of aging. Now we know better. Although a small amount of physical decline is natural, most of the loss comes from disuse. At this Milestone, body comp isn't primarily about looking good in your Levi's. It's about living free and independently.

After menopause, around age 52, the typical woman starts losing a pound of muscle a year. Remember—a pound of muscle burns about 35 to 50 calories per day. If you drop 3 pounds of muscle, you lose the power to burn up to 150 calories a day. Yet you continue to eat as though you still had the muscle, which results in a 15-pound weight gain in 1 year. There's no mystery here—just math. So when you let your muscle tissue slide, you're inviting fat to come in. And in this Milestone, the more muscle you lose and the more fat you gain, the less you'll be able to do for yourself. And we're not talking about scaling Everest. We're talking about showering, cooking, bending, and cleaning. Plus, as we discussed earlier, the fat you gain at this time of life doesn't pad your hips and butt; it can fill the inside of your abdomen, where it raises your risk for heart disease and diabetes.

The good news is that physical activity has a huge effect on these body composition changes. The esteemed Fels Longitudinal Study, which investigated aging, body composition, and lifestyle, found that physical activity had profound effects on body composition in postmenopausal women. Postmenopausal women who ramped up their physical activity—doing intense activity like running, fast cycling, or fast swimming several times a week—weighed up to 26 pounds less than did nonathletic women and had markedly less body fat.

If you remember our rule of thumb, strength training becomes even more important during this Milestone and could even help shave off Toxic Fat. One study found that when women strength-trained three times a week for 16 weeks, they lost significant amounts of belly fat. Plus, they got more than 50 percent stronger. Sounds like a bargain to me!

Think it's too late to start exercising to improve body comp? Never! Resistance-training expert Miriam Nelson, Ph.D., has reported that postmenopausal women could increase their strength by 35 to 77 percent in 12 months if they lifted weights just twice a week.

## WHAT'S HAPPENING IN YOUR HEAD

In this Milestone, change is constant—and it can be stressful. Children move away and start lives of their own. Friends and loved ones fall ill and pass away. Maybe you have some health issues yourself. This is no time to stick your head in the sand. It's a time to stick your chin out and practice stress resiliency, which I discuss in part 3. Once you learn to regroup, life in this Milestone can be fulfilling and satisfying, even throughout periods of sometimes-stressful change.

Many women in this Milestone worry about experiencing mental decline and developing dementia and Alzheimer's. Alzheimer's affects two to three times as many women as men; it's been hypothesized that this difference between women and men may be related to estrogen loss as well as to the quality of lifestyle. (Of course, it may also be because women live longer.) But studies show that exercise—both physical and mental—can keep your gray matter sharp no matter what your age.

When David Snowdon, M.D., did his famous Nun Study of 94 sisters of the Notre Dame order, ages 77 to 99, he showed how these vital, resilient women—many of whom have gone on to become centenarians—stayed physically and mentally active throughout their lives. Their rates of Alzheimer's were much lower than that of the general population. The reasons: good nutrition, regular physical activity, and the ability to shed stress. They embraced life to its fullest. But they also spent a lot of time reading and writing in their journals, something that other studies have pointed to as the kind of mental exercise that will keep your brain humming along healthfully. One study even found that people who read books or did puzzles and played board games on a daily basis were less likely to get Alzheimer's than were those who didn't.

Don't fret about becoming the old woman you never wanted to be—there's little danger of turning bitter and bent if you keep up your activity and maintain a healthy body comp. Researchers from the University of Wisconsin have reported that women over age 60 who exercise regularly are more satisfied with their lives and happier in general than are women who do not exercise. I've worked with hundreds of women in their sixties, seventies, and even older, and I'm here to tell you that it doesn't have to be that way. Over and over, I've seen women step up to the plate and live this Milestone with passion and zest. You can, too.

## YOUR BIGGEST HEALTH CHALLENGES

There's no question that years of using our bodies results in some wear and tear. Expect medical conditions to emerge. Instead of feeling helpless, hopeless, and defeated about any physical limitations you may have garnered, learn to adapt and work around them. Here are the health issues you'll want to keep an eye on in Milestone 4.

**Battle aches and pains.** If you've got a bum knee from when you were overweight or from years of running, the answer isn't to sit out the rest of your days. Tell yourself, "In the midst of difficulty lies opportunity." Find an activity that doesn't hurt your knee. How about water aerobics, or restorative yoga? Can't run? Ride a bike, swim laps, or take an indoor Spinning class. The key is to show yourself that you can adapt to change. Those women who do, live life to the fullest.

**Keep your bones sturdy.** Estrogen helps protect your bone mass. After menopause, your body hits the fast-forward button on bone loss. That makes osteoporosis a major public-health threat for more than 28 million Americans, 80 percent of whom are women. A staggering one in two women over the age of 50 will have an osteoporosis-related fracture in her lifetime. But the last thing you should be doing is sitting back. Countless studies have shown that weight-bearing exercise like walking, running, and lifting weights can help keep your bones strong.

When French researchers recently studied 56 women ages 60 to 81, they found that the stronger a woman's quadriceps (the muscle on the front of the thigh), the stronger her femur (thighbone). Likewise, researchers at the University of Florida found that when postmenopausal women strength-trained 3 days a week for 24 weeks, they increased bone strength by almost 2 percent—an increase that can mean the difference between a bruise and a break if you take a spill.

**Heads Up!** Share your Mind-Mouth-Muscle experience. Research shows that the larger your group of friends, and the stronger your connections and sharing with them, the longer and more joyfully you live. Start with your own family. Got sisters, daughters, granddaughters, cousins, or nieces who want to share a meal or take a walk with you? Find other Milestone 4 women and join them for travel, walks, bike rides, meals, and just plain hangin' out. There's power in sisterhood. Here's a grand opportunity to put your Mind-Mouth-Muscle into action. The reward is more health, love, and joy to go around.

YOUR CUSTOMIZED HEALTH SOLUTIONS

At this Milestone, to stay engaged in life, you have to contribute to life in some meaningful way. Now this may sound ironic—first I tell you to take time for yourself, and now I advise you to give your time freely. Why? Because it'll keep you connected—to your family, to potential friends and opportunities, and most of all to yourself.

### Mind

I live by Helen Keller's call to arms: "Life is either a daring adventure, or nothing at all." There's no reason you can't push the envelope of aging in your own special way.

**Go back to the school of life.** Learning is a lifelong process, and the more you learn, the more you grow and the younger you stay. Start checking out classes at the community college. If you ever wanted to know more about growing prizewinning vegetables, brush up on your piano playing, or learn more about modern art, this is your chance. Think active, movement, play.

**Maintain your social network.** The landmark Nurses' Health Study, which examined more than 56,000 women ages 55 to 72, pointed to the importance of social contact. One of the strongest predictors of functioning well through this life Milestone was having close friends and/or relatives. Most remarkably, women who were part of a close social network not only tended to be healthier and happier but also recovered more quickly from diseases of all kinds, including heart attack, stroke, and cancer. Among centenarians studied, attending church or other spiritual services provided essential social contact as well as what they called a "life-enhancing" ingredient to their existence. Consider investing in a computer so you can correspond with distant friends or relatives. With the prevalence of e-mail and adult education centers and activities, as well as church and travel groups, there is no excuse to live your life alone.

### Mouth

Because your digestive system can be less efficient as you get older (meaning you don't necessarily digest all the nutrients you need), make every bite you take as nutrient-packed as possible. Cut back on—or eliminate—the white starches, like rice, potatoes, and pasta, and replace them with colorful vegetables and fruits, which have tremendous nutritional value. Also, you'll want to <u>watch your portion sizes</u>. During this Milestone, fat tends to account for a greater percentage of your weight, which reduces the number of calories you burn—and need. Follow the Body-*for*-LIFE for Women Eating Method in part 4, along with these special tips for Milestone 4.

<u>Go for color.</u> During this Milestone, you may notice that you're content to eat less frequently and stick with main meals and an afternoon snack. You may eat less at dinner, too, especially after age 65. You may also be more comfortable eating dinner earlier, as you'll probably be going to bed earlier than in previous Milestones. You're adjusting to changing physical activity as well as physiological changes in your tastes and interest in food. This is all normal and natural.

When you do eat, <u>concentrate on fruits and veggies that have a deep, rich color. They have the highest levels of antioxidants, minerals, and vitamins.</u>

**See red.** Though all fruits and vegetables are good for you, studies suggest that you should find a special place on your plate for the red ones, like tomatoes and watermelon. In the University of Kentucky Nun Study, researchers found that 70 percent of those with the highest levels of blood <u>lycopene, an antioxidant found in red fruits and vegetables</u> (especially tomatoes), were still alive 6 years later, compared with only 13 percent of those who had the lowest levels of blood lycopene.

**Mind your nutrients.** We all know folks who take a pharmacy's worth of vitamins, minerals, and herbs every day. Guess what—centenarians don't have to lay down their life savings at GNC. <u>All you need is a basic multivitamin that includes vitamins $B_6$, $B_{12}$, and D</u> (your body may not be able to absorb these important vitamins like it used to) and a few additional supplements. These are:

- Omega-3 fatty acids (1,000 milligrams taken twice per day)

- Vitamin E (400 IU) to help prevent heart disease and cancer

- Selenium (100 micrograms) to help prevent heart disease and cancer

- Calcium (1,200 to 1,500 milligrams a day if you're 51 or over) for bone maintenance

- Coenzyme $Q_{10}$ (100 milligrams a day) for heart and brain health
- Folic acid (800 micrograms) to help lower the risk of several chronic, degenerative diseases

## Muscle

In Milestone 4, there are no ifs, ands or buts about it. You must move every day to maintain a healthy body composition and stay vibrant and active—and, most important, to stay independent and out of the hospital. Strength training may be the most important exercise for women in this Milestone. Studies by my good friend Dr. Miriam Nelson show that even women in their nineties can reap the benefits. However, you'll need to adapt the Body-*for*-LIFE for Women Training Method to fit your personal health and fitness level. If you can swing it, consult a personal trainer who specializes in training older women (you can find them in senior centers and Ys everywhere), and follow the special tips for Milestone 4. The great news is that there are now more trainers who are women over 50 and who are experienced in working with Milestone 4 women. You'll find them at your local YWCA or community center.

**Follow the 5-minute rule.** If you do nothing else, get up and move for 5 minutes every hour. This is especially true if you have any disabilities that limit your mobility. Maybe it's walking the perimeter of your yard. Maybe it's taking a walk up and down the stairs. Could even be cleaning out your closets. This is what I call slow-drip exercise. You don't need to set aside a big block of time, and the benefits add up. Think about it: If you move 5 minutes an hour for 9 hours a day, you've sneaked in 45 minutes of exercise.

**Do your own chores.** As you get older, you'll likely find plenty of well-meaning friends, relatives, and neighbors willing to rake your leaves, carry your groceries, and sweep your sidewalks. Unless it's a task you really can't handle—like shoveling wet, heavy snow—tell them thanks but no thanks. The more daily chores you can do on your own, the stronger your body will stay and the more independent you can remain.

**Give gentle exercise a try.** There are countless varieties of gentle, nonimpact exercise that women in Milestone 4 can enjoy, from water aerobics to restorative yoga and tai chi. These activities improve balance, stamina, flexibility, and coordination, which translates into a higher quality of living. Tai chi has also been shown to reduce the pain of arthritis, and there are even special videos you can buy, like *Tai Chi for Arthritis,* so you can work out at home.

**Stretch it out.** I don't have to tell you that we get less flexible with every Milestone. But all you need to do to stay limber is incorporate the stretches in Appendix A into your daily activity. The best time to stretch is when your muscles are warm. So before you stretch, do 5 to 10 minutes of light exercise to get your blood flowing.

## YOUR MILESTONE, YOUR PROGRAM, YOUR BODY-*FOR*-LIFE

So now you've learned how a woman's unique physiology affects not just her overall health and risk of disease but also her ability to maintain a healthy weight. I've used the new findings in the field of gender-specific medicine—based on the newest science—to create a blueprint that can help any woman get fitter and leaner and stay healthy, now and in the future. Now we're ready to drill deeper into the specifics of the plan. In the next few parts of this book, I'll introduce you to a female-friendly way to navigate the stresses that can affect a woman's ability to achieve her Body-*for*-LIFE (Mind), a female-centric way of eating (Mouth), and a for-women-only formula for physical activity (Muscle). Ready? Let's go!

# Mind: The 10 Body-for-LIFE for Women Power Mind Principles

## Part 3

*"It's not the team that wants to win, that wins. It's the team that wants to win, and is willing to work at it, that wins."*
—Vince Lombardi

I can close my eyes and picture the scene perfectly: I'm meeting with a patient for a follow-up visit. As she settles into the overstuffed armchair across from my desk, I can see that she's anxious and upset. I know what's coming—I can see it in her eyes. I brace myself for these six little words: "I was doing really well until . . ."

You've probably said them yourself, dozens of times. You know the drill. You're doing great, eating right, getting in your daily workouts, and something happens. You hurt your back or shoulder and find it difficult to train. You move to another town, change jobs, begin or end a relationship. Maybe life just gets crazy and suddenly you're overwhelmed and lost, missing workouts and turning to food for comfort. By 4:00 P.M., you're up to your ovaries in stress and your motivation is gone. The hell with mini-meals and lean protein. What you need is a pile of cookies.

I sympathize, ladies—I've had my share of these days from hell. But life happens, and life is about adapting to whatever shows up at your door. I have no doubt that you're a master at helping the people you care about get through tough times. But when things get funky in your life, do you give yourself the same treatment? Who gives you the big pat on the back when you rescue yourself?

Body-*for*-LIFE for Women is all about turning that feminine impulse to nurture inward and becoming your own best caregiver, despite whatever obstacles life places in your path. In part 1, you made a commitment to doing just that, and you owe it to yourself to persevere, come hell, high water, PMS, an argument with your honey, endless deadlines, or a kid covered with chickenpox. And you can stay the course. Because though you can't always control those challenges, *you can choose how you will respond to them.*

That's why Body-*for*-LIFE for Women emphasizes mental transformation as the foundation for physical change. If you are to achieve and maintain a stronger, healthier Body-*for*-LIFE, you must have the mindset for success. A mindset that allows you to cope with Toxic Stress along with all the other demands of a woman's life, while continuing to care for yourself. I call this mindset Power Mind.

Women with Power Mind have learned to:

- Handle stress in positive ways rather than resort to overeating, abusing alcohol, smoking, or other self-destructive behaviors

- Balance caring for themselves with caring for others

- Do the work it takes to achieve their goal of mind-body transformation

- Anticipate and work around life's speed bumps that interfere with their self-care

- Get their self-care back on track when they get stuck

One of my favorite maxims is "In the midst of difficulty lies opportunity." I don't see mistakes—I see opportunities to learn. Open your heart to the lessons. If you view challenging life events as opportunities to recommit to your self-care, rather than as overwhelming obstacles, you will overcome them. These Power Mind Principles will help you stay on track when life gets tough.

## PRINCIPLE 1: EMBRACE ADVERSITY

You've had it. You're tired of feeling like crud every day, and you're determined to get in shape—mentally and physically. Chances are, something has happened in your life to put you in this state of readiness. You're so tired that a front-end loader

**Principle 1 Tool: The Contract with Yourself**

In part 1, I invited you to take the Body-*for*-LIFE for Women Pledge. Well, this Tool is the Pledge, in contract form. Yes, I want you to put your intentions in writing. On the best stationery you can find—no scrap paper—I want you to write this out (or photocopy) and complete the following contract to yourself.

Date: _____

I _____, commit to starting my Body-*for*-LIFE for Women program on _____ (date), completing this 12-week Weight Removal (or Maintenance) Segment on _____ (date). I believe that I can accept and complete my Challenge to the best of my ability.

I realize this is work and accept the self-care price I must pay to achieve my mental and physical transformation.

I commit to keeping my daily Mind-Mouth-Muscle Journals.

I will practice the 10 Power Mind Principles to help me stay the course.

I will expect and adapt to adversity and embrace tough times as learning opportunities.

I will strive to take action and not to ruminate, bitch, moan, or whine.

I commit to pursuing progress, not perfection, in my eating and training.

I will find joy to neutralize my stress, take my Mini Chills, and strive to become a master regrouper.

I will be self-assertive and fight for the right to take care of myself.

I will acknowledge and reward myself for my achievements along the way.

By completing the Challenge, I signify honor and respect for myself, and affirm that I deserve health, happiness, and joy.

Place your contract in a plastic page saver and hang it in a prominent place (maybe the refrigerator?) to refresh and renew your commitment. Renew your contract after the completion of every Weight Removal Segment.

couldn't get you up in the morning. Maybe your partner made a comment—gentle or otherwise—about your funky moods or your appearance. Maybe you just came back from the mall empty-handed because nothing fit—again—or from the doctor, who lectured you about your rising weight, blood pressure, cholesterol levels, and blood sugar. Perhaps you've watched in envy and amazement as a friend, family

---

**The Rule of Reverse Expectations**

As you embark on your Body-*for*-LIFE experience, live by the <u>Rule of Reverse Expectations</u>: *Anticipate that there will be obstacles in your path*. When you encounter them, embrace them as <u>opportunities to learn to stay the course with your eating and training</u>.

---

member, or colleague changed their unhealthy ways, removed a ton of weight, and then ran their first 5-K for charity. Whatever—something inside you clicked (or snapped). You're ready to change—no, transform—and that's very good news.

Hold on. I know you're filled with hope, energy, and anticipation. I know you're willing to do whatever it takes because the pain of staying where you are far outweighs the pain of the work it will take to change.

But if your positive changes are to be permanent, you must adopt the Rule of Reverse Expectations. It goes like this: *Anticipate that there will be obstacles in your path.* Then, when you meet up with them—and <u>it's not a matter of if, but when</u>—you'll greet them as opportunities to sharpen your skills at keeping your self-care on track. <u>Instead of getting frustrated by those obstacles, embrace them.</u> Remember that in the midst of difficulty lies opportunity. <u>Identify the opportunity and the lesson hidden in that obstacle, rather than obsessing about the obstacle itself.</u>

So your gym is closed because the roof fell in? Walk or run outdoors. Your partner is complaining that you spend more time with your dumbbells than with him? Invite him to join you. In each instance, you have an opportunity to allow adversity to make you a stronger, wiser woman.

I once had a patient named Carla, a bright and beautiful lawyer who was undergoing treatment for breast cancer. During one appointment, she said to me, "You know, my cancer has taught me a valuable lesson. While I was driving to your office today, I got caught in a traffic jam. Instead of getting bent out of shape, I put on a CD, kicked back, and simply enjoyed the music. <u>I just don't see the point of getting angry anymore. I've learned to savor every minute of my life."</u> Wise woman, that Carla.

With the Rule of Reverse Expectations, you <u>relish, rather than run away from, the challenge of self-care. You stop simply talking about eating right and working out regularly, and actually do it.</u> You are armed with realistic expectations, a doable program of self-care, and the Power Mind to stick with your plan.

You will do battle with your inner demons that try to pull you back into your familiar, self-destructive ways. You'll have good days and funky ones. But in the end, you'll win. Every single time you embrace the Challenge, you win; you're that much closer to the best woman you can be. (See "Principle 1 Tool" on page 59.)

## PRINCIPLE 2: FIND YOUR MOTIVATIONAL "BULL'S-EYE"

When I was in medical school, I was taught that the greatest motivation to change an unhealthy lifestyle stems from the desire to prevent or treat a disease. Surely a woman who's just had a coronary bypass would get a clue and change her unhealthy ways, right? Wrong. I still carry with me the vivid memory of a woman I sent packing after a four-vessel bypass, who told me she couldn't wait to load up on her favorite fast food and light a cigarette to celebrate. My lesson was to reexamine this whole motivation issue.

Over the years, I've come to realize that much of the time—maybe even most of the time—getting healthy simply isn't enough of a motivation to change. I know how counterintuitive this sounds, but it's true. You see, every day there's this divide between your A.M. intentions and your P.M. realities. I call them your A.M./P.M. motivations. In the A.M., you wake with hope in your heart—fully intending to take care of yourself—or the fear of developing heart disease, diabetic complications, or lung cancer like your mother or aunt did. Funny how by 4:00 P.M. that hope or fear doesn't keep you from eating the M&M's on your colleague's desk or going through an ashtray for cigarette butts. If it did, you'd be fit and healthy or smoke-free by now.

So why the disconnect? Perhaps denial has something to do with it. Could it be that you really do snack too much, plop on the couch a bit too often? Or that you could quit smoking but just don't want to? Hey, I'm not here to make you feel bad. I'm here to help you to blast through the denial. To hold your nose and cannonball into the dark place of raw, gut-level truth. To get real about some very tough issues that, upon closer examination, cause you pain. As the folks in recovery groups say, pain is the touchstone of progress. So diving into that place of pain—that I-just-can't-take-it-anymore place—is actually a healing and very courageous first step.

Think of motivation as a target, the kind used in archery. A standard archery target

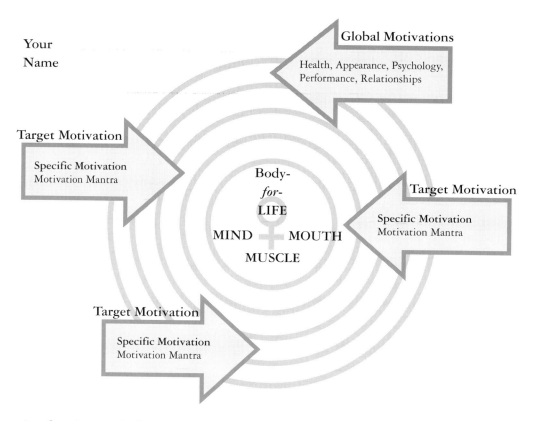

has five rings and a bull's-eye. You, ladies, are aiming for your Motivational Bull's-Eye—the motivation that resonates most powerfully for you. I've developed a three-step process for hitting it.

1. **Develop your Global Motivations.** The outermost ring of the Motivational Target (the one farthest from the bull's-eye) contains your Global Motivations—your general reasons for wanting to become fitter and healthier. Typically, Global Motivations fall into one or more of the following categories.

- Health: You want to prevent and/or treat a health condition.

- Appearance: You want to become fitter and more attractive.

- Psychology: You want to develop more confidence, optimism, and self-esteem.

- Performance: You want to improve your physical body or mental outlook.

- Relationships: You want to develop more positive and intimate connections at home, at work, and in the world at large.

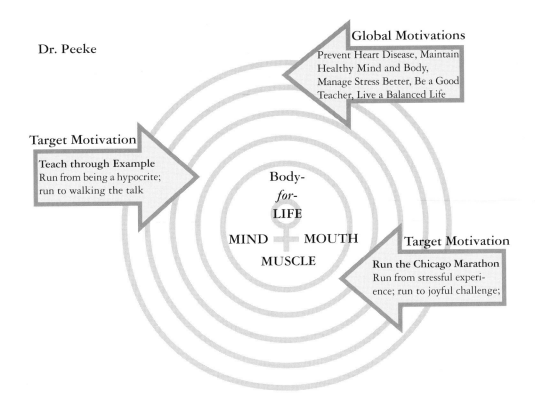

**Dr. Peeke**

**Global Motivations**
Prevent Heart Disease, Maintain Healthy Mind and Body, Manage Stress Better, Be a Good Teacher, Live a Balanced Life

**Target Motivation**
**Teach through Example**
Run from being a hypocrite; run to walking the talk

Body-
*for-*
**LIFE**
**MIND** ⚥ **MOUTH**
**MUSCLE**

**Target Motivation**
**Run the Chicago Marathon**
Run from stressful experience; run to joyful challenge;

What are your Global Motivations? To feel energized? To prevent obesity or disease? To remove weight and get fit? To feel better physically and mentally? To fit into a certain size again? Whatever they are, write down at least three in a notebook that you will use throughout your Challenge. Remember—they're *personal* motivations, so there are no "wrong" answers.

1. _____

2. _____

3. _____

These Global Motivations are a sturdy foundation upon which your Target Motivations can develop. But while they're admirable, they often don't pull at your heart or your gut enough to get you through the afternoon or evening, which are prime overeating hours. They don't resonate at the moment you need them—the moment

**Principle 2 Tool: Create Your Motivational Target**

Drawing out a Motivational Target serves two purposes. First, it reveals your true motivations for wanting to change—the reasons that go beyond fearing death or disability. Second, you're forced to think about what matters to you—what imbues your life with joy and meaning. Typically, the exercise takes 15 minutes or less—so little time for so much return. Here's how to do it.

Sit down with a piece of blank white paper. Draw an imaginary archery target—at least four rings and a bull's-eye. Ask yourself one question:

*"Why do I want to change my body?"*

Write down the first three answers that come to mind.

Chances are, they represent your Global Motivations: *I want to change because I want to be healthier. I want to change because I'll die if I don't.* Whatever your answers, distill them to simple phrases so that they're easy to recall. Then write them inside the outermost ring.

Let's go deeper now. Ask yourself again:

*"Why do I want to change?"*

Get real personal. Search your mind for answers that stop you in your tracks. I don't care what they are—everything's game here. Your answers might be deep and serious or witty and humorous.

Again, write out the first three answers that come to mind. These are likely to be your Target Motivations. Boil down each one to a key phrase and devise a Run-From/Run-To Motivational Mantra. Write it in the bull's-eye.

Place this paper inside a plastic sleeve and leave it on the passenger seat of your car. Each time your motivation is threatened, move through the rings until you find the Motivational Bull's-Eye that keeps you on course at that particular moment. And don't forget this exercise each time you feel that your motivations have changed.

when your hand is on the refrigerator handle, or at the end of the day, when you're on the fence about whether to change into your sneaks and sweats or simply go home. Enter the Target Motivations.

**2. Identify your Target Motivations.** When the power of your Global Motivations peters out—and it will as the day goes on—you'll proceed to the inner rings of your Motivational Target, which contain what I call your Target Motivations. They're the "why" in this whole journey you're taking, beyond your health and perhaps even your vanity. They're deeply, deeply personal. They get at why you're doing the Challenge at all, and why you're doing it now. It's critical for you to really dig to find what's driving your efforts, because those motivations will see you through the tough times. You'll know when you find your Target Motivations, because you'll feel a *click* deep in your soul. Examples of a Target Motivation:

"I want to prove to myself that I can follow through on something."

"I'm tired of hating myself—I want to love myself as much as I love my family."

"I want my kids to be proud of me."

The key is in the *click.* Just close your eyes, repeat it to yourself, and wait to feel that sense of resonance, the feeling that makes your stomach flip a little, when you know something speaks to you. If you mentally try out a Target Motivation like this and it clicks—that is, it's powerful enough to keep you motivated, focused, and on track—then whammo! You've hit the bull's-eye! Use it until it no longer clicks; then move to the next Target Motivation to see if it hits your bull's-eye.

All right, let's give it a whirl. What are your Target Motivations? Write down at least three.

1. _____

2. _____

3. _____

**3. Create a Run-To/Run-From Mantra for Each Target Motivation.** As you identify each Target Motivation, anchor it with a Mantra that will conjure up its power when you're feeling most beaten up, overwhelmed, and frustrated. The Mantra should be simple, contain a powerful visual image if possible, and smack you in the head like an invisible two-by-four so it will snap you out of your "I gotta eat" trance. It should also contain the phrases "run from" and "run to."

Here's an example of how you might come up with a Mantra.

You buy Oreos for your kids and your partner, and they love them. But having the

*(continued on page 68)*

### The Motivational Bull's-Eye in Action

Amanda, 45, wanted to remove the 40 pounds she'd accrued over the past 5 years of 100-hour workweeks; mothering Susan and Shelley, her teenage girls; and caring for her parents, whose health was declining. Here's how she and I hammered out her Motivational Target. She started off with typical motivations to change.

## GLOBAL MOTIVATIONS

1. Reverse high blood pressure.

2. Get off cholesterol medications.

"Good start," I said. "But apparently, it's not enough to stop you from hitting the Oreos when you get home from work."

She tried again. "I want to feel better," she said. "I'm sick of being stressed-out and exhausted and fat."

## GLOBAL MOTIVATIONS

1. Manage stress in positive ways.

2. Gain more energy.

"Fine," I said. "But are these enough to get you on the treadmill at 6:00 A.M. or make it to your yoga class? Let's dig deeper. What in your life gives you joy?"

"My daughters," she said.

"Of course," I said. "And what gives *your* life meaning?"

After some pondering, she said, "What gives my life meaning is being a great mom. Teaching my daughters how to live well."

"Now we're getting somewhere," I said. "Back to the question. *Why do you want to change?*"

"I want balance in my life, and I want to show my daughters how to stay balanced, too. I don't want them to be like me, stressed-out, overweight, and struggling."

"Hmm," I said, and then added gently, "So, what are you telling Susan and Shelley when you don't go to yoga class, and get home so stressed-out that you blow through a pint of Häagen-Dazs? Can you go a little deeper? What about you? Think of yourself now. Why do you want to change?"

Amanda spent a full minute considering this question. And then she said quietly, "Because I want to love myself as much as I love my family. Because I deserve that love. I'm a good person, and I deserve to live as long and as well as I can."

Bull's-eye. Amanda had formed her first set of Target Motivations.

## FIRST RING

Motivation: To love and honor myself

Mantra: *Run from* neglecting my body and mind; *run to* identifying and satisfying the people, events, and things that bring me joy

## SECOND RING

Motivation: To be a great mom

Mantra: *Run from* abandoning daughters; *run to* mentoring Susan and Shelley

## THIRD RING

Motivation: Lose perimenopausal back roll

Mantra: *Run from* back roll; *run to* backless dress

## FOURTH RING

Motivation: Hike a mountain with my daughters

Mantra: *Run from* fatigue and joylessness; *run to* being fit and powerful

Amanda drew out her Target and referred to it every day. To reinforce her Motivational Bull's-Eye, she kept a picture of her daughters on her computer screen saver, on her desk at work, on her nightstand, and on the refrigerator door. She also put small photos inside the kitchen cabinet doors, to remind herself to stay on track. It showed her exactly why she chose to eat nourishing food and make it to yoga class and hop on her treadmill so early in the morning.

Six months later, she'd finished two segments of her Challenge, and brought her daughters to my office to meet me. She looked fit and joyful, proving once again that women who make the right choice look it.

cookies in the pantry causes a peck of trouble for you. You have two choices: to eat them or not to eat them. What you have to do is imagine the consequences for each of these choices.

If you eat them, what is the consequence? This consequence has to really bother you, and the vision you conjure has to take away your appetite. How about this: You're standing in the hot summer sun, dressed in dark, shapeless clothing that feels more like a shroud. You're sweaty and uncomfortable as you watch others jog in shorts, bike in colorful clothes, enjoy life. So "sweaty shroud" is what you run *from*. What do you want to run *to*? After thinking long and hard, you might conjure up a vision of yourself on a bike, clad in a pair of clingy biking shorts and riding up a long hill on a country road. You look and feel fit and free. You're joyful, happy, loving life. Okay. You got it.

Target Motivation: To be happy, fit, and free, living life to the fullest.

Motivation Mantra: *Run from* sweaty shroud; *run to* bike ride on country road, feeling joyful and free.

Are this Motivation and this Mantra powerful enough to help you stay the course? The only way to know is to try them. (For an idea of how one of my patients came up with her Target Motivations and accompanying Run-From/Run-To Mantras, see "How Terri Found Her Motivation—And Mantra.")

Repeat this three-step process for each of the inner rings. You'll end up with at least four Target Motivations, any one of which can function as your bull's-eye.

If you've ever hit a plateau and found it difficult to muster up the motivation to continue with your weight-removal program, consider this: Your original Target Motivation may no longer be powerful enough, and you may need to replace it with a new one. For example, perhaps you're back on the bike and can now pedal with the best of them. Great. Now, perhaps your Motivational Bull's-Eye will be to take on a daylong or weekend biking tour with a group. As you achieve your goals, the Target Motivations have to change because you've changed—you've removed a significant amount of body fat, say, or increased your fitness level—and you're ready for new challenges. Identify those new Target Motivations, allow them to challenge and invigorate you, and you'll always stay fresh and on course.

## How Terri Found Her Motivation—And Mantra

At 5 feet 5 inches and 190 pounds, Terri had flown in from five states away to meet with me. This 45-year-old high school teacher had hopped on and off every diet and was mystified as to why she couldn't stick with any of them.

As it turns out, Terri didn't lack motivation. She had simply misidentified it. She thought her motivation to change was her family history of heart disease and her climbing cholesterol. But that Global Motivation couldn't keep her from eating a huge serving of pasta at night.

"To find your Target Motivation, you have to dig deeper," I said. "If that candy is in front of you and you really don't need it, or haven't planned it as a treat, you have two options: to eat it or not to eat it. For each of those two options, there is a consequence. That's where your Target Motivation and Motivation Mantra are hiding."

As we talked, Terri came to see that her greatest joy in life was to teach her children and students to take better care of themselves. But she couldn't do this unless she could inspire not just with words but with actions. The messenger—Terri herself—had to be as powerful as her message.

If she didn't eat the cookie, she was a Teacher. If she did succumb, she was, in her words, a Hypocrite.

"Which do you want to be: Teacher or Hypocrite?" I asked. Whammo! Motivational Bull's-Eye and Mantra, right there in front of her. One choice gave her joy. The other acted like an appetite suppressant. Now she was armed to duke out her demons from 3:00 P.M. on.

As Terri journeyed through her Weight Removal Segments, she realized that the more she stuck with her Target Motivation, the more she fulfilled the goals of her Global Motivation—her cholesterol plummeted, along with her body fat and her risk of heart disease.

Terri's Motivational Bull's-Eye—to be that superb and inspirational Teacher—is enough to help her fight her demons, at least for now. One of her Target Motivations—to start running again, which she'd done in the past and loved—was also a strong driver, just not enough to stop her from overeating during her vulnerable hours. But perhaps one day, when Terri feels that she's achieved her goal as a great Teacher, she'll focus on training for her first 5-K—and find her next Motivational Bull's-Eye.

## PRINCIPLE 3: JOY YOURSELF

When I first meet a patient (or meet the group of women on my Peeke Week Retreats), one of the first questions I ask is this: What in your life gives you joy?

Typically, women answer, "My partner" or "My kids." Of course, I reply. But aside from your family, what gives you joy? Too often, their reply to that question is a blank stare.

Although caring for a family is indeed rewarding and joyful, it's only one aspect of what makes a woman whole. To be truly fulfilled, she must discover what brings her joy outside of caregiving, whether that's returning to school, starting her own company, writing, growing a garden, or cooking gourmet meals. Then she must integrate this joy into her life. Until she does, it will be all but impossible for her to sustain her self-care.

I remember Anna, a wonderful 54-year-old woman who was diagnosed with terminal colon cancer. Her family and friends encouraged her to quit her graduate studies in psychology—which gave her much joy—and take a cruise around the world. She didn't particularly want to, but she didn't want to disappoint the people who loved her, either. After all, they were thinking of her, weren't they? So she booked the cruise.

Anna lasted about 3 days and then flew home. In those 72 long hours, she'd discovered that what really brought her joy was being among her loving family, tending her enormous rose garden, and continuing her graduate studies. From then on, Anna made it a point to define her joys and to pursue them with energy and passion. She endured her therapies and continues to live joyfully.

I use "joy" as a verb. I like to remind my patients to pay attention to daily joys by asking them, "So—have you joyed yourself lately?" They proudly respond with stories about their new puppy, their first-ever 5-K walk, the bouquet of daisies they bought for themselves, or a yoga retreat.

To bring joy into your life, you have to believe you deserve it. Most men, feeling entitled to happiness, defend their joy time (think *Monday Night Football,* Friday-night poker games, hours hammering and drilling at the garage workbench). Not so women. Well, that's got to change. Go for it. Get out there and joy yourselves.

---

**Principle 3 Tool: Joy Yourself**

Taking this test can help you home in on the things that give you joy—or the things that might, if you gave them a chance.

Each time you're confronted with a demand on your time, ask yourself this question:

*"Will including this thing, event, or person in my life ultimately bring me joy?"*

**If you answer "Absolutely!":** Chances are, you're about to engage in an immediate joy—planting your garden, catching up with your best friend over coffee, taking the day off to chaperone your child's field trip. Congratulations—you've discovered what brings you joy during your brief time on this planet.

**If you answer "I don't know":** Give that thing, event, or person a whirl. You may find that, say, herbal body wraps make you claustrophobic. Okay, no joy there. But how about discovering that your new book club is filled with interesting women who spark your brain? Score one for joy! Don't be afraid to experiment—get out there and play.

**If you answer "No":** Then why would you allow this thing, event, or person to be a part of your life? You might not be able to completely eliminate it from your life, but you can limit the amount of time you devote to it. Do that, and you'll preserve the joy you already have and protect yourself from things that detract from it.

---

You also have to be willing to put in the work to find joy. (See "Principle 3 Tool.") New joys come into the lives of the women who seek them. I never knew the joy of running until, at the age of 40, I laced up my sneakers and gave it a try. Now, as I write this book, I'm in training for my third marathon. Who knew?

## PRINCIPLE 4: BITCH, MOAN, AND WHINE, BUT GET THE JOB DONE

On a small end table, next to the armchair that my patients sit in during their appointments, sits a ceramic jar labeled "Dr. Peeke's Early Retirement Fund." Whenever a patient starts in with the negative self-comments, she has to put a dollar into the jar. At the rate some of my patients put themselves down, I'll be playing golf 24/7 in no time.

---

**Principle 4 Tool: Dig Yourself Out of the Rumination Rut**

To control the BMW (Bitch, Moan, and Whine) that keeps you in the Rumination Rut, make it a habit to patrol the inside of your head for negative thoughts that make you feel helpless, hopeless, and defeated. When you find one, shout (out loud if you're alone, silently if you're in public), "*Stop!*" Then immediately replace the negative thought with a self-nurturing statement. Say something that you might tell a good friend struggling in the same situation. Here's an example.

*BMW:* "I can't do this program anymore. My muscles are killing me. I feel like a loser in front of those gorgeous young things at the gym. What's the use? I might as well park myself in front of the tube and eat. I've lost 10 pounds, but I still look like a sack of potatoes."

*Nurturing statement:* "Look, finding the time and energy to fit in my self-care will always be a challenge, and some days will be better than others. But that doesn't mean it's impossible. It's work, but what worthwhile project isn't? I have more energy, I'm down a dress size, and I really am making progress! I'll just do the best I can and celebrate the days I can really rock to it."

See the difference?

Now, whip out your Body-*for*-LIFE for Women Pledge from part 1. Study it. Recommit to action rather than rumination. Repeat after me: "I will no longer *think* about getting fit and joyful. I'm gonna *do* it—today!"

---

Look, girlfriends—you can't change your life if you're busy engaging in self-abuse. Listen to yourself sometime: "I'm stupid, I'm fat, I'm ugly, I'm a failure, my legs are too short, nobody wants me. . . ." Would you allow your child or a dear friend to talk about herself like that? Not likely. Besides, such trash talk is useless. All it does is mire you more deeply in the Rumination Rut.

In the dictionary, the first definition of *ruminate* is "to go over in the mind repeatedly." The next definition is "to chew repeatedly for an extended period." Let's see, stewing and chewing in response to stress—boy, did Webster get that right! When women fall into the Rumination Rut, they mentally stew over the same worry or problem until they're emotionally drained—yet they've solved nothing. While they're stuck in this negative mindset—which can last a day, a week, or a year—their regular walks or workouts, healthy eating, and regular checkups fall by the wayside. Not coincidentally, so does their zest for life.

Working with thousands of women—and men—has shown me that compared with men, women are far more likely to ruminate about how unattractive and unfit they are, rather than create a plan of action; more likely to berate themselves for a binge, rather than try to regroup and figure out why it happened so that it won't happen again; more likely to worry about how they look in their workout gear, rather than to learn the correct way to do a dumbbell fly.

Once you're in the Rumination Rut, you're vulnerable to BMW—bitching, moaning, and whining—about your body, your willpower, your behind, your this, your that. The more you do the BMW thing, the deeper you dig yourself into the Rumination Rut. It's a vicious cycle.

The biggest source of BMW-ing is refusing to accept that achieving and sustaining your mental and physical transformation takes work. That's right—mental and physical sweat, intensity, mindfulness, focus—all the things, by the way, that you apply to your job, your kids, and your relationships. Why shouldn't you expend the same energy on yourself? Humbly accept that your self-care will take work, and you'll make the journey so much easier.

To gain control of BMW and to drag yourself out of the Rumination Rut, you've got to break its hold. Employ any distraction technique at your disposal: Get off the couch and go for a walk. Take the kids bowling or roller-skating. Clean out your closets. Do anything but let your brain hold your butt hostage. (See "Principle 4 Tool.")

## PRINCIPLE 5: SHOOT FOR PROGRESS, NOT PERFECTION

Some women have a huge problem with this principle because all their lives, they've tried to be perfect—the perfect wife, the perfect mother, the perfect employee, the perfect friend. How about you? Will you try to be the perfect Body-*for*-LIFE success story, too? I sure hope not, because this program is not about achieving perfection. It's about achieving a mental and physical *transformation.* It's about optimizing your strengths, navigating around your vulnerabilities, and goin' for it.

In 2001, at the White House, I met Nadia Comaneci, the Romanian gymnast who achieved a perfect score at the 1976 Summer Olympics. She was sitting next to me as we viewed the premiere of a documentary on women in sports. I commented on her amazing career and her "perfect 10."

I'll never forget her reply: "My scores were perfect because they were numbers," she said. "I, however, am not perfect. I'm a human being."

There can never and should never be perfection in a living thing. There's nothing human about perfection, nothing to endear or inspire. When a great athlete stumbles, we gasp. But we cheer when that athlete picks herself up, re-groups, and succeeds on the next try. To strive is human, and it's the essence of Power Mind.

Look, no woman—no human being—eats and trains perfectly day after day, year after year. So striving for perfection is a prescription for endless guilt, and guilt is as useless as rumination. More important, guilt eats away at the positive energy you need for making progress and feeling joy, leaving you instead feeling defeated and empty. If you're too terrified to take that first step for fear of not being perfect, you'll go nowhere. Perfection, therefore, leads to paralysis, not progress.

"Progress, not perfection" means that if you work hard and keep your focus 80 per-cent of the time, you're doing great. The other 20 percent of the time, you get to be human—fallible. Are you in the grips of hormonal mayhem today? No worries. Blow off your workout today. You'll regroup and bounce back tomorrow. If you fall off the wagon for a day, a week, or a month, and binge, don't carry on like the world is coming to an end. Look for the lessons. Figure out why that binge occurred so it doesn't happen again; regroup, and get back on track.

One of the best ways to live by this principle is to fill out your daily Mind-Mouth-Muscle Journals. Reflect on your day and write down three things that you did well and that helped you move forward. This gives you positive reinforcement and helps you build momentum because you're giving yourself credit where credit is due.

And cut yourself some slack here, ladies. Quit spending your time ruminating on why your day didn't go "perfectly." Instead, adjust your expectations and celebrate every little accomplishment, no matter how small. (See "Principle 5 Tool.")

---

**Principle 5 Tool: Shoot for Progress, Not Perfection**

Instead of saying "I aim for perfection," say "I aim for progress."

Instead of saying "I wasn't perfect," say "I did the best I could, given the constraints and restrictions in my life."

Every time you feel the urge to say *but,* say *and* instead. Consider the difference:

"I removed 20 pounds and I'm more fit, *but* I have another 15 pounds to go and I still run too slow."

"Yes, I removed 20 pounds and I'm more fit, *and* I'm progressing well with my self-care."

You nip perfection in the bud *and* give yourself a powerful and loving affirmation. Way to go!

---

## PRINCIPLE 6: DON'T LET STRESS GO TO YOUR HEAD— OR TUMMY

For most women, stress is a constant companion. It's there as they speed to work, pay the bills online, pick up a gallon of milk at 10:30 at night so everyone can have their cereal the next morning. In one survey on stress conducted by the National Women's Health Resource Center, nearly 93 percent of the 681 people surveyed described the level of stress in their daily life as moderate or higher. Fewer than half said they always felt capable of coping with it—that's a lot of un-coped-with stress floating around.

There are two main categories of stress in a woman's life. First, there's everyday stress, something I call Annoying but Livable Stress. This includes your standard stresses—the daily commute, the parking ticket, the computer malfunction—along with the stresses that arise from major milestones, like getting married or having a child. This kind of stress, we expect and should be able to manage.

Toxic Stress, on the other hand, leaves you constantly overwhelmed and drained. It grinds you down day after day, year after year. It erodes your immune system and makes PMS and perimenopause a living hell. It also ramps up your appetite for comfort foods and can pack on pounds of fat deep inside your tummy, expanding your girth and making you more vulnerable to heart disease, diabetes, and cancer.

**Principle 6 Tool: Don't Let Stress Go to Your Head—Or Your Tummy**

Photocopy at least 10 of my handy dandy Stress Rx signs (see opposite page and page 78). Tape the first sign ("The answer is not in here!") onto your fridge, kitchen cabinets, pantry—even on the vending machine at work, if you dare. (Who knows—folks might even appreciate the gentle reminder.)

Tape the other Stress Rx sign ("The answer is in here!") to your workout bag or dumbbells in your home gym, your bath salts, your favorite relaxing CD, your treadmill, your favorite herb tea, or your phone.

When you confront that first sign, close your eyes for a second. Ask yourself, "What am I running *from* right now?" Pause. Acknowledge and accept your pain and allow it to pass through you. Then take a deep breath and say, "The answer is not in this fridge/vending machine/pantry/shop."

Now walk quickly toward what you know will soothe that pain—your workout gear, treadmill, phone. Ignore the familiar, seductive voice inside your head that shouts that food is what you need, or that you're too fat to be seen in the gym. Listen to that relaxing CD, call a member of your Estrogen Squad (see Principle 10), sip a mug of your favorite tea. Be with your feelings. Honor that new voice inside you. It's the voice of empowerment, and each time you withstand stress in a positive way, it will become louder and stronger.

Work is a huge source of Toxic Stress for women—perhaps the biggest. In one study, 60 percent of employed women cited stress as their number one problem at work. In another study, of more than 21,000 nurses (the ultimate caretakers), Harvard researchers concluded that on-the-job stress weakens a woman's health as much as smoking or a sedentary lifestyle. And when they get home from these stressful jobs, women must take care of their families. They're always doing for and giving to others, which leaves them little time or energy to do for or give to themselves.

Your real holy grail is the quest for balance in your rich and challenging life. Stress is manageable when you take even a little time to neutralize the mental and physical price of eternal caregiving. A manicure, a pocket of peace to nap or just hide in a corner and read, a good laugh with your best friend—it doesn't take a month in a spa to achieve sustained de-stressing.

STOP!

# THE ANSWER IS NOT IN HERE

**Stress Overeating Rx:**

**Instructions:** Photocopy this page and tape it to your refrigerator, pantry door, snack drawer, office refrigerator—anywhere Junk Carbs beckon when you're stressed.

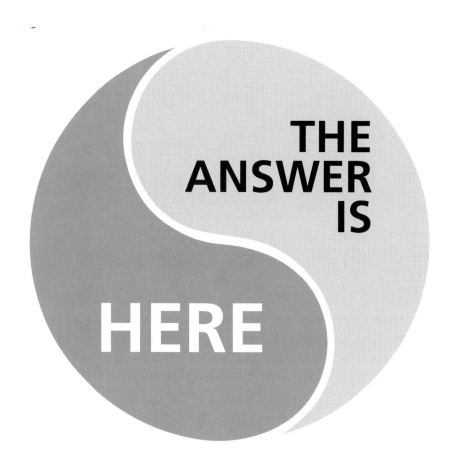

**Stress Overeating Rx:**

**Instructions:** Photocopy this page and tape it to your treadmill, workout bag, bath salts—on anything that helps you honor your commitment to self-care.

There's a Chinese proverb that states, "Tension is who you think you should be. Relaxation is who you are." Take a deep cleansing breath and think about that for a moment. Isn't it true? The bottom line is that Toxic Stress will rapidly age you, make you fatter, and increase your risk of dying early. There's a better way, a simple way for you to short-circuit your impulse to overeat, even when you're staggering under a boatload of stress. (See "Principle 6 Tool" on page 76.)

## PRINCIPLE 7: GIVE YOURSELF A LICENSE TO CHILL

Buddha said: "We are what we think. With our thoughts, we make the world." But if you're in a continual state of depression, anger, frustration, or fatigue, your world will feel pretty small and unfulfilling. That's why I want you to commit to investigating relaxation techniques and then commit to practicing one.

Meditation, yoga, tai chi, progressive relaxation—it doesn't matter which you choose, as long as you like it and practice it regularly. I recommend that you take a class, but if you can't, buy a book or video. Taking a class serves three purposes: You get correct instruction, meet other like-minded people, and automatically build some "me" time into your day. (But if you can't, simply turn to "Principle 7 Tool" on page 80.)

Meditation is one of my favorite relaxation exercises. Taking time to meditate each day gives your mind an opportunity to chill out, to take a break from fretting and obsessing and ruminating. Ideally, you'll meditate for one extended chunk of time—say, 10 to 20 minutes—and do 5-minute mini-meditations throughout the day.

Research supports meditation's positive effects on mood. What's more, it appears to literally change the minds of those who practice it. In a study published in 2002 in the *Journal of Psychosomatic Medicine,* brain scans of new meditators who were guided in meditation 3 hours a week for 8 weeks showed significant increases in activity in a part of the brain associated with positive emotion. What's more, the heightened activity persisted for at least 4 months after the experiment, when the study participants were scanned again.

If you've never practiced a relaxation technique, you may feel strange—perhaps even a bit overwhelmed—when you stop all the frantic activity to simply sit still. Be

**Principle 7 Tool: Give Yourself a License to Chill**

When you need tranquility now, try this simple technique.

Find a quiet, comfortable place where you won't be distracted.

Sit with your back straight. Place your hands in a comfortable position.

If you wish, call on God or a higher power to help you.

Allow your eyes to rest comfortably downward, gazing softly but not focusing on anything. Let your breathing become deep and rhythmic.

It's okay to let your attention drift a bit, but stay relaxed. If your eyes become heavy, let them close. Don't worry about doing it right. You simply want to clear your head and relax.

Although you can do this exercise throughout the day whenever you feel the need, it works even better if you do it for 10 or 20 minutes, once or twice a day.

You might also try "walking meditation." It's just what it sounds like—combining a walk with quiet reflection. Don't focus on a destination—with walking meditation, it's the journey that counts. I call it "medicating with movement." You use your own brain chemicals—endorphins and serotonin—to soothe yourself, boost your mood, and just plain feel better.

To try walking meditation, simply turn your full attention to the movements that make up the act of walking. Really break down this most basic of acts. For example, as you lift each foot, silently say to yourself "Lift." As you move your leg forward, say "Move." Then say "Step" as you place your foot on the ground. The more you focus on these movements, the calmer you'll feel.

patient with this process—and above all, give yourself a chance to work through any discomfort you may feel. Eventually, you will come to depend on your relaxation technique not just to relieve stress but to delve more deeply into your self. (See "Principle 7 Tool" and the relaxation tool on page 35 for two options.)

## PRINCIPLE 8: LEARN TO BE A MASTER REGROUPER

To regroup is to practice your self-care the best you can in the worst of circumstances. To regroup means that no matter what hits you, you accept and adapt to life's challenges without engaging in self-destructive habits. The ability to regroup allows you to continue a healthy eating and activity plan no matter what the crisis.

Regrouping comes down to learning how to move from Plan A to Plan B—or to Plan Z, if that's what it takes. A woman's natural tendency is to become paralyzed once Plan A no longer works. But regrouping is a dynamic process requiring constant tweaking. The goal is to keep regrouping until you achieve a new plan that works for you. Your "Plan Me."

Plan A is your life on schedule. You eat breakfast every day at 7:00 A.M., you walk on your lunch hour, you have your "me" time every night after 9:00, after you put the kids to bed. Plan A goes seamlessly about once a year. I encourage you to relish the moment.

Plan B is your life on stress. You've been up all night with your youngest, who has a nasty bout of stomach flu, so you're sleeping when you usually eat your egg-white omelet. You're under the gun at work, so the big report takes precedence over your walk. Your mom and sister are having another one of their interstate wars, so you've been on the phone with one or the other every night, instead of cozying up with a book or dropping, semicomatose, into a bathtub. In the midst of this hailstorm of stressors, how do you tend to your self-care?

You go to Plan C, D, E . . . and finally Plan Me.

One of my patients, Samantha, a TV news producer, pretty much had to regroup her way through the alphabet. In a 6-week period in 2003, her husband tripped over the family dog and fractured three ribs, her 9-year-old daughter was diagnosed with attention deficit disorder (which required the scheduling of multiple specialists for testing), and her mother, who lived one state away, fell and broke a hip, which required Samantha to visit each weekend. The coup de grâce? The Iraq war broke out and her work schedule became 24/7. I was exhausted just listening to her.

Clearly, her Plan A was useless. For each event, she shifted to a new plan, tried it out, and refined it until it became her Plan Me. One of her secrets to success was learning to call upon others for help and support. Her group of friends (her "Estrogen Squad," as I like to call them) helped care for her family while she worked ridiculous hours at the television studio. Her husband, now housebound, tutored her daughter when she was unable to. She filled the office refrigerator with Smart Proteins, Carbs, and Fats—cheese sticks, mini-containers of cottage cheese, fruit, single-serving packages of almonds (we'll talk about this more in part 4, Mouth: The Body-*for*-LIFE for Women Eating Method). And whenever she could, she walked around the office or neighborhood to de-stress and stay as fit as she could under the circumstances. It might not have been the gym, but it was something, and that something kept her from stress overeating and piling on boatloads of weight.

To commit to regrouping, you need to believe that you're worth your own time, and that while you can take pride in caring for others, it takes a really strong, balanced, healthy woman to care for herself. I've taught my Peeke Performers to regroup, and these ladies are now quite macho about it. They have turned the tables on stress management and, using their Power Minds, shout, "Go ahead, Peeke. Stick me in

---

### Principle 8 Tool: Learn to Be a Master Regrouper

Write down what your healthy eating and activity plan would look like on a low-stress day. That's your Plan A.

Now make a list of everything that could wreck that plan: an illness, a deadline, a needy friend or family member, a broken treadmill. Now rewrite your Plan A, incorporating any of these problems and devising ways to work around them. Create Plans B, C, D, and E. Here's an example: It's too cold to take your Plan A walk. Go to Plan B—walking in the mall or on the health club's treadmill.

How to regroup after falling off the wagon? Say to yourself, "Okay, things got a little nuts. Now I've got to get back to Plan A." Or if Plan A is no longer possible, create a new Plan A. Give yourself 3 days of withdrawal and regrouping to regain momentum. In these 3 days, you'll refocus on Plan A, practice it, and let it gel before diving in with full steam.

**Day 1:** Plan how and when you'll eat and exercise. Squash the BMW! Keep busy, and get to bed early. It's a scientific fact that you can't eat and sleep at the same time. Opt for the sleep.

**Day 2:** Repeat Day 1. Congratulations! You made it without indulging in any self-destructive behavior or BMW. Get to bed early.

**Day 3:** Repeat Day 2. By now, feelings of accomplishment should be making you feel more in control. Good for you! You've just proven my favorite saying: In the midst of crisis is opportunity. You'll think twice before you allow yourself to go off the deep end again.

any situation. I'll show you how I'd handle it without dropping the ball." (See "Principle 8 Tool.")

## PRINCIPLE 9: FIGHT FOR YOUR RIGHT TO SELF-CARE

I often watch as women try to get their partners and family to help them enough so that they can create time for their self-care. Meeting resistance, they throw up their hands and simply give up. Not anymore. With Power Mind, you stand your ground and make it work, one way or the other. You realize that you're not being selfish. You're just asking for balance.

I've got news for you. No one is going to book your gym time for you. No one is going to shop and buy chicken breast and grill it for you. And no one is going to offer to watch the kids while you work out at the gym, then treat yourself to a matinee. If you don't plan and do it, it isn't going to happen.

First, develop your own mission statement using the "Principle 9 Tool" on page 84. Knowing your mission teaches you to establish boundaries, draw a line in the sand, and say, "This is my time, and I'm here to defend it." You're on your treadmill and the phone rings. That's why God made voice mail. It can wait. Your self-care can't.

To cure a chronic case of "yes-itis," here's what to do the next time you're asked to do something that you can't or don't want to do.

1. Ask yourself, "Will saying yes further my mission statement?" For example, if you've already volunteered for countless PTA fund-raisers in the past year, do you really need to take on another? Must you show up for a neighborhood meeting on selecting flower beds for the subdivision entrance?

2. If the answer is no, say in a calm and caring tone, "I'm so sorry, but that doesn't work for me right now. Maybe next time."

Wow. Saying this shows that you know what does work for you. Now, once you've said it, stick to it. Stand up to anyone who tries to argue you down. Keep your refusal courteous but definite, short but sweet, and don't get into a lengthy debate.

Okay. Let's review. What will you say the next time your son, daughter, or anyone else interrupts your run on the treadmill to talk about something that doesn't involve the loss of a limb?

---

**Principle 9 Tool: Develop Your Mission Statement**

Every successful company has formulated a mission statement—a paragraph or two that states the company's reason for being: why it exists, whom it serves, and what it hopes to achieve. A mission statement will help you determine the limits and boundaries of your time and energy, and how you should "spend" your efforts in life.

Here's how to create your own.

Write down no more than 10 sentences that describe what you want to accomplish in your life and what is important to you, both personally and professionally. For example:

I, _____, aspire to be the best mother, spouse, and daughter I can be. I commit myself to providing love and support to my dear ones throughout my life. I am grateful for the gifts I was born with and will strive to use them to help myself as I help others. I also commit to honoring my intellectual, physical, and spiritual needs, following through on my daily obligations, and providing my company with the best work I can do.

You can now take anyone's request of your time, quickly compare it with your mission statement, and see if there's a match. If there isn't, say "I'm sorry. I can't [insert request here]. It doesn't work for me right now. Maybe next time."

---

"I'm sorry, honey, but that doesn't work for me right now. Let's talk about this right after I finish in 20 minutes."

Ah, sweet music to my ears—and it will be to yours, too.

## PRINCIPLE 10: FORM YOUR OWN "ESTROGEN SQUAD"

Research shows that people trying to make healthy lifestyle changes are more likely to succeed when they have a strong support network. With a minimum of effort, you can assemble your very own Estrogen Squad.

That's not to say that your support system can't include men. But in my experience, women tend to be better at giving one another the love, nurturing, and support they need as they struggle to honor their commitment to self-care. You'll call one or more members of your Estrogen Squad when you're about to do something self-destructive—like blow off your workout or embark on a binge—or

## Principle 10 Tool: Form Your Own Estrogen Squad

In the middle of a blank piece of paper, draw a large circle and label it You. Now draw four other circles around "You" and label them Family, Friends, Professionals, and Other.

Now, inside each circle, write the names of one or more women who you feel could be included. (In some cases, the circle might be empty—that's fine.) For example, in your Family circle, you'd choose one or more members of your immediate or extended family with whom you'd feel comfortable sharing your deepest feelings. Your circle might include your mother or sister, a special aunt, maybe even your teenage daughter. If you think they might like to join the Challenge with you, all the better.

Do the same for the Friends circle, choosing the one or two women who have given you the most support and encouragement and who might like to join the Challenge with you.

Do the same for the Professionals circle. Here you might include a personal trainer, your therapist, or your family doctor, if he or she is caring and supportive of your goals.

Finally, repeat the exercise for the circle labeled Other. These folks might include a sympathetic acquaintance you've met in a yoga or tai chi class, a local support group, or a weight-removal chat room, or it might be someone from your place of worship.

As you fill in each circle, remember that you needn't come up with 20 names. Three or four women will be plenty.

Once you've assembled your Estrogen Squad on paper, you can approach them (or a select few) in person, by phone, or by e-mail. Explain that you're embarking on the Body-*for*-LIFE for Women Challenge, and that one of the exercises in the book requires you to form a support system. Then ask them if they'd be willing to offer support and advice, say, once a day for 10 minutes. (This assures them that you won't forever be crying on their shoulder.)

How many self-generated sources of support were you able to find? Chances are, more than you thought!

One more thing: You have to work at maintaining your Estrogen Squad. As with tending a rose bush, you have to be mindful and pay attention to its needs. Trust me—the blossoms are worth every ounce of sweat.

you'll seek their perspective if you find yourself neck-deep in the Rumination Rut.

Your Estrogen Squad could be one person, 10, or anywhere in between. As with food, it's not quantity that counts—it's quality. To assemble your Squad, look in the following four groups: family, friends, professionals, and support groups.

From your inner circle, choose one or two people you most depend on, with whom you feel comfortable sharing your deepest feelings—your mother or sister, a special aunt, maybe even a teenage daughter or son. Then choose the one or two friends who have given you the most support and encouragement in your quest to achieve a healthier lifestyle, or who might like to join the Challenge with you. Professionals might include a personal trainer, a therapist, or your family doctor, if he or she is caring and supportive of your goals. (If not, look for another physician who is. That's part of self-care, too.)

Finally, you might round out your Squad with a sympathetic acquaintance you've met at work, or someone from your place of worship.

The people in your Squad should be kind, of course, and willing to share their precious time with you. They should also be able to look you straight in the face and tell you that the dress doesn't work for you, or that you're making everyone nuts with your endless BMW-ing. A sassy sense of humor never hurts, either.

A woman's Power Mind works best when supported by her assertive, witty, loving, and nurturing sisters. Armed with her Estrogen Squad, a woman will see her quest for mental and physical transformation become a reality. (See "Principle 10 Tool" on page 85.)

## NOW YOU'RE READY

As I've said before, the Mind portion of the Mind-Mouth-Muscle formula is the cornerstone of the entire Body-*for*-LIFE for Women plan. You're now ready to move on to the nitty-gritty details and learn how to eat and train to create your best Body-*for*-LIFE.

If you should lose your footing along the way, please come back and review these pages. You know the answers are in here, and inside of you.

You have the power. Use it!

# Mouth: The Body-for-LIFE for Women Eating Method

## Part 4

*"Instead of eating carelessly and hurriedly, in the midst of noise, agitation, and arguments, and then going off to do yoga exercises, wouldn't it be much better to understand that meals give you the perfect opportunity every day, two or three times a day, to practice relaxation, concentration, and the harmonization of all the cells of your body?"*
—Omraam Mikhael Aivanhov, *Golden Rules for Everyday Life*

Now we're ready to tackle the second component of the Mind-Mouth-Muscle Formula: Mouth (a.k.a. the Body-*for*-LIFE for Women Eating Method). This discussion can't come a moment too soon because the only way to finally achieve your Body-*for*-LIFE is to get off the dieting treadmill.

Fad diets are like hemlines: They're up, they're down, but they always come back. And though they may be dressed up a little, they're essentially the same: They deprive a woman's body of the food and nutrients it needs, and women themselves of the pure, primal pleasure of eating. And when these diets fail—which they inevitably do—women despair. They feel helpless, hopeless, defeated. Studies show that women on restrictive diets have abnormally high stress hormone levels, which eventually leads to stress overeating and weight regain. This makes me crazy because it's so completely preventable.

Throughout a woman's life, eating takes on many different meanings. When you were a little girl, it was fun. No calorie counting, no obsessing about fat content. Just real ice cream, a lump of heaven in your sugar cone. The teen years brought training bras, curves, and PMS carb cravings. Young adulthood turned stress overeating into a second career. Pregnancy and the family thing make self-care a mission impossible. By perimenopause, our closets start to look like Filene's Basement, with 10 sizes reflecting years of stress-eating roller coasters. Managing a healthy weight has devolved into an endless, vicious cycle of quick-fix, science-fair-project "diets" followed in a desperate effort to battle the shock of bodies that no longer feel like our own.

There is a better way.

When the original *Body-for-LIFE* swept the country, its dietary message was simple: The low-fat, high-carbohydrate diet recommended by so many nutrition experts, and riddled with processed sugars and starches, makes you fat. The human body works best when it's fueled by a balance of carbohydrates and protein. Later, in *Eating-for-LIFE,* published at the height of the low-carb frenzy, Bill Phillips expanded upon that message: Don't be so quick to condemn carbohydrates.

I agree. The fact is, male or female, the human body needs carbohydrates. They're the body's preferred source of fuel. The brain's, too. That's why when you don't eat enough of them, you soon begin to feel draggy, irritable, depressed, and fuzzy-headed. You haven't given your brain the fuel it needs! Your body, either. The bottom line is that carbs alone are not the only reason for overweight.

Here's the thing: Eating the right balance of carbs and protein is especially important for women. When women learn to fuel their bodies the correct way, they drop body fat and build shapely muscle—regardless of their ages, how much weight they have to remove, and their impossible schedules.

The Mouth portion of the program—the Body-*for*-LIFE for Women Eating Method—is effective because it factors in a woman's unique body composition (the body's proportion of muscle to fat), her unique nutritional needs, and the demands of her high-stress, overcommitted lifestyle.

To get the astonishing results that you see on the inside cover of this book, you have to follow this way of eating (and the exercise portion of the program). But you can't do that unless you believe, really believe, that your health and happiness are worth pursuing.

You don't have to wake up dreading another day of wearing dark and shapeless clothes that hide your body. You don't have to be tired or depressed all the time. I know that any woman of any age can change her body—and her life—once she learns how to nourish herself, both physically and mentally.

I urge you to read the next section on your nutritional needs, broken down by milestone. But if you're raring to go and want to jump in right away, you can turn to page 93 and begin at "Smart Women, Smart Food Choices."

## YOUR NUTRITIONAL NEEDS, MILESTONE BY MILESTONE

Over the course of their lives, women ingest 50 million calories. That's equivalent to 18 tons of food. You need to spend those calories wisely.

As a woman, you need more of certain specific nutrients than men do. For example, throughout their lifetime, a significant percentage of women don't consume enough calcium, so they come up short as they approach menopause, when shifting hormones naturally decrease bone density. In your childbearing years, you need more iron to prevent iron deficiency anemia, a significant health issue for women in Milestones 1 and 2. (Menstruation and pregnancy affect blood levels of iron.) And both before and during pregnancy, women need extra amounts of the B vitamin folic acid to protect their unborn children from birth defects.

The sooner in life a woman begins to eat well, the better—and the Mouth principles of eating are so well-balanced that it's the optimal diet for most women, regardless of age. Let's look at a woman's unique nutritional needs—and challenges—through the filter of her hormonal Milestones.

### MILESTONE 1: MENSTRUATION THROUGH FIRST PREGNANCY

These years in a young woman's life are often chaotic. She's pulling all-nighters, working odd hours, partying. . . . She's going, going, going. So she skips meals or eats on the run—usually processed and fast foods, which shortchange her of critical nutrients. USDA research shows that fewer than half of young women get even 50 percent of the recommended amounts of most vitamins and minerals—including calcium and iron, which are particularly crucial for young women. The teen years and early adulthood are the most critical for building good bone density.

How women in Milestone 1 eat now may have a significant effect on their ability to conceive or to maintain a healthy weight in general. Overeating fat- and calorie-packed processed and fast foods often leads to overweight or obesity, which can adversely affect female fertility and pregnancy. It may also lead to nutritional deficiencies that can set them up for health problems down the road.

But some young women have the opposite problem: In relentless pursuit of the "perfect" bodies they see in magazines and on TV, they don't eat enough—or at all. Severely restricting calories, as in anorexia, or bingeing and purging, as in bulimia, deprives a woman's still-developing body of the vitamins and minerals it needs for growth and optimal health. Untreated, eating disorders can have grave physical consequences.

The challenge for women in Milestone 1 is to find a nutritional middle ground, neither gorging on junk nor drastically curtailing fat or calories. It's that balance issue again. The Mouth part of the Body-*for*-LIFE for Women plan provides a balance of protein, carbohydrates, and healthy fats. It's also brimming with fruits, vegetables, and other plant foods, which contain health-promoting, disease-fighting compounds: antioxidants, vitamins, minerals, fiber, and phytochemicals.

**Heads Up!** Don't make the mistake of thinking that you can eat junk now and make up for it later. It might not be as easy as you think, especially if you start to gain weight in this Milestone and don't manage to remove it. A study conducted in 2004 showed that if a woman carries even 20 extra pounds from her early twenties into adulthood, her risk for breast cancer rises.

## MILESTONE 2: THE REPRODUCTIVE YEARS

Most women in this Milestone are at their peak—Mother Nature planned it that way. These are the "double-, triple-, and quadruple-shift" years. Although the years of child rearing and career building of this Milestone can be among the most joyous and fulfilling of a woman's life, they're often the most stressful. To take it all on and keep going strong, women in Milestone 2 must fuel their bodies with top-notch food.

Some women savor their independence and choose not to have children. For them, managing their Milestone 2 health and weight gain gets a bit more challenging than in Milestone 1 but, with regular exercise and proper attention to nutrition, is entirely doable.

Other women start their families in this Milestone. It's best to conceive after you've nailed healthy eating, maximized your fitness, and done what you can to keep your body fat in the 25 percent range. If you haven't yet had children but plan to someday, the rule is to eat today as if you'll conceive tomorrow. You know a woman's diet has a significant impact on her fertility. Although the Body-*for*-LIFE for Women Eating Method assures women of getting many of the nutrients they need, women in this Milestone who are planning a pregnancy should take a daily multivitamin supplement that contains 400 micrograms of folic acid. Women who get this amount before they conceive and through their first trimester slash, by half, their risk of delivering a baby with birth defects like spina bifida.

Many pregnant women, frightened by the prospect of spending the rest of their lives in stretch pants, try to gain as little weight as they can. But mothers-to-be who skimp on food while they're pregnant can inadvertently cause a host of problems for their babies later in life. Low birth weight can contribute to a baby's risk of chronic diseases later in adulthood, including diabetes, obesity, high blood pressure, and heart disease.

On the other hand, pregnancy isn't an excuse to balloon to the size of a Hummer. Excessive weight gain raises the risk for gestational diabetes, which can cause health problems for both mother and child. (If you're pregnant, follow your doctor's dietary advice. After delivery, and especially if you're nursing, ask your doctor if the Body-*for*-LIFE for Women Eating Method is appropriate for you.)

**Heads Up!** If overweight or obesity runs in your family, pregnancy may bring out a genetic vulnerability to weight gain, even if you have never had a weight problem. Work with your doctor to stick to the recommended 25 to 35 pounds of weight gain—your Milestone 3 body will thank you.

## MILESTONE 3: PERIMENOPAUSE AND MENOPAUSE

I hate to be the one to deliver the bad news, but after having broken it to thousands of women, it seems to be my lot in life. Here's the deal: If you've been winging your diet up to this point, the winging is over. From this point on, to stay at a healthy weight and an optimal level of body fat, you have to pay attention to what, how much, and how often you eat. Period.

In this Milestone, most women soften up from their belly button to their pubis. The result? The menopot, an accumulation under your skin of 5 to 10 pounds (depending on your height) of fat, which lies on top of your abdominal muscle. This weight gain is natural and caused primarily by fluctuating levels of the female sex hormones estrogen and progesterone. Though fit women gain the minimal amount of fat, most of them gain it nonetheless.

There are two rules to live by in Milestone 3. Rule one: Eat right and get active to minimize your menopot. Rule two: Fight like heck not to put on weight. Once you gain those extra pounds, they're murder to get off.

By following the Mouth eating guidelines, you'll get all the nutrients that a Milestone 3 woman needs while you help stave off excessive weight gain. I can't promise you that it will get you back into the jeans you wore in college. But I can assure you that if you're overweight, this way of eating will help you remove a significant amount of body fat. You'll also minimize the stress eating and carbohydrate cravings that seem to plague women in this Milestone.

**Heads Up!** If you haven't yet cleaned up your diet, you're getting to last call. Beginning with this Milestone, a woman is at increased risk of developing age-related chronic diseases—cardiovascular disease, osteoporosis, diabetes, and cancer. The Body-*for*-LIFE for Women Eating Method is your customized nutrition prescription. It's low in saturated fat (the artery-plugging kind found primarily in animal products, such as meat and dairy) and moderately high in heart-protective monounsaturated fats, and packed with cancer-fighting fiber. Fiber can also improve your body's sensitivity to the hormone insulin and therefore help prevent diabetes. The plan's ample amount of fruits and vegetables provide a natural source of "health insurance": antioxidants. These substances—which include vitamin C, beta-carotene, and plant substances known as phytochemicals—are believed to lower a woman's risk of heart disease, cancer, Alzheimer's disease, and stroke.

## MILESTONE 4: BEYOND MENOPAUSE

If you've hit this Milestone, you should continue to eat well to reduce your risk of age-related diseases. And that means what it means in every Milestone: minimizing or eliminating processed sugars in your diet, and choosing lean proteins and healthy carbs and fats in appropriate portions to accommodate your postmenopausal metabolism.

The Body-*for*-LIFE for Women Eating Method meets your needs by providing the blueprint for appropriate amounts of lean protein and, of course, those disease-battling veggies, fruits, and whole grains. Let's not forget about water. As women age, they tend not to get as thirsty. So pay special attention to drinking enough of it. (You won't forget—it's one of the Body-*for*-LIFE for Women Eating Method principles, as you'll see.)

**Heads Up!** Stay sharp by packing away those fresh fruits and vegetables. The New England Centenarian Study at Harvard Medical School, as well as the Nun Study, showed that a diet rich in fruits and veggies helps reduce the risk of Alzheimer's and dementia and contributes to longevity.

## SMART WOMEN, SMART FOOD CHOICES

When Bill Phillips wrote the first *Body*-for-*LIFE,* the country had just emerged from its love affair with fat-free foods. We all learned the hard lesson about the folly of stripping every gram of fat from our diets. The truth is that there are unhealthy fats (which I call Junk Fats), and then there are the fats that are good for us—the Smart Fats.

Smart Fats are the monounsaturated fats in healthy foods like nuts, grains, avocados, and olive oil. Junk Fats are the saturated and trans fats. Saturated fats are primarily in animal foods, such as in fatty meats, butter, and whole-fat cheese—hence my insistence on lean proteins like fish, chicken breast, and low-fat dairy. Trans fats hang out in foods made with or cooked in hydrogenated vegetable oil, restaurant-fried foods, margarine, and processed cookies, cakes, crackers, and snack foods. Trans fats have been shown to be more health damaging than saturated fats—they raise "bad" LDL cholesterol while they lower "good" HDL cholesterol. (Thankfully, food manufacturers will be required to list trans fat on product labels by January 2006, which means they're scrambling to remove trans fats from their products now.)

The same thing happened after the country's whirlwind romance with low-

### Stress: The Formula for Female Fat

In my first book, *Fight Fat after 40,* I linked women's constant, unremitting stress, which I dubbed Toxic Stress, to a predictable hormonal reaction that can lead to weight gain in all women, but especially in women over 40. I called this reaction the Stew and Chew Response.

Our prehistoric sisters experienced a different kind of stress than we do today—the stress that came with trying to survive in a hostile environment of razor-toothed predators. They experienced the fight-or-flight response, which existed to gear up our bodies to fight the threat or, well, to flee from it. Today women experience no such threats to their survival. But assaulted by chronic, unremitting stress, their bodies have the same fight-or-flight reaction.

But women don't fight. They don't flee. They *eat.* Essentially, the Stew and Chew Response is the 21st-century woman's version of the fight-or-flight response. And it's not just the calories from those stress-induced cookie frenzies that pack the weight on. Women are done in by their own hormones.

Here's the Cliff's Notes version of what happens. Chronic stress triggers the adrenal gland to produce a flood of cortisol. This stress hormone signals the liver and bloodstream to release their stores of fuel, called glucose, to cope with the imminent "emergency." Maybe the emergency is watching your son take a spill on his skateboard without his helmet, or trying to meet a crushing deadline. Cortisol also travels to the fat cells located inside the tummy. Once there, it convinces them to give up fat to fuel the stress response.

So there you are, stressed out of your mind, with all that sugar and fat floating around in your bloodstream. Your body is waiting for you to use this energy. But because sitting and stewing doesn't take all that much effort (and I'm talking about *physical* effort), your cortisol levels remain high.

But wait: It gets worse. This prolonged secretion of cortisol triggers the flow of the hormone insulin. Insulin facilitates the storage of fat, especially fat that settles around the midsection. It also triggers cravings for fat and carbohydrates—sometimes uncontrollable cravings. That's why, like a moth to a streetlight, you gravitate to high-fat, high-carb foods, like doughnuts and chips.

Funny how tuna on a bed of greens never quite does it for a woman stressed out of her brain at 10:00 P.M. If she's anything like me, she's more in the mood for a ménage à trois—her, Ben, and Jerry.

carb dieting: We learned to distinguish between Smart Carbs, like sweet potatoes and oatmeal, and Junk Carbs, like cupcakes and white bread. The press started throwing around terms like "good fats" and "bad fats," "good carbs" and "bad carbs."

But here's the deal: I don't use "good" and "bad" to describe food. It might seem nitpicky, but I have a good reason for feeling the way I do. I've worked with too many women who used those terms to describe what they ate, and almost all of them equated eating "bad" food with being a bad person. You eat "bad" foods like a doughnut or a few slices of pizza, you feel bad about yourself, you feel hopeless and helpless about your body, and your Toxic Stress increases. Thus begins the vicious cycle of stress overeating, depression, and Toxic Fat.

So instead, I use different shorthand: Smart Foods and Junk Foods. Smart Foods are made up of Smart Fats, Smart Carbs, and Smart Proteins. Smart women eat Smart Foods.

Of course, the food we choose does have an impact on our health and our dress sizes. And though we all know to limit the Junk Foods, the real challenge is to eat the appropriate portions of the Smart Foods. Because eating too much of any food, Smart or otherwise, will increase your body fat and your odds of getting heart disease, diabetes, or cancer.

Junk Carbs—think anything made with white sugar and white flour—are particularly detrimental to a woman's health. Two recent studies suggest that a diet high in Junk Carbs raises a woman's risk for two kinds of cancer. In one study, researchers from the National Cancer Institute looked at data from the 18-year Nurses' Health Study and found that sedentary, overweight women who eat diets high in added sugar and white flour have a 53 percent increased risk of pancreatic cancer, a particularly deadly form of cancer.

The second study looked at the diets of more than 2,500 Italian women with breast cancer and an equal number who were cancer-free. The findings: The women with breast cancer were eating more foods high in refined carbs. These types of foods—white bread, white pasta, packaged baked goods and snack foods—boost blood sugar and insulin levels and trigger a rise in the insulin-like growth hormones linked to breast cancer risk.

Finally, if you eat a lot of Junk Carbs, chances are that you're missing out on fiber. Don't care about your health? Well, it turns out that fiber is important for weight loss, too. A Harvard study showed that over the 12-year study period, women with the lowest intake of dietary fiber gained an average of 3 pounds more than did those who consumed more whole grain fiber. In an important study conducted at Tufts University, a team of researchers reviewed several weight-loss studies and discovered that adding an extra 14 grams of fiber to your diet each day leads you to eat 10 percent fewer calories a day. That means if you normally eat 2,500 calories a day, you might automatically cut down to 2,250—which would lead to a removal of 2 extra pounds a month!

## THE MOUTH FORMULA AT WORK: THE BODY-*FOR*-LIFE FOR WOMEN EATING METHOD

The whole Body-*for*-LIFE eating philosophy can be summed up in one sentence.

**Eat the right foods, in the correct amounts, at the right times.** So it's all about quality, quantity, and frequency. If you follow these principles for the next 12 weeks—and beyond—you'll remove excess body fat; build feminine, shapely muscle; safeguard your bones; and support your ultimate goal: to live long and well as a mentally and physically powerful woman.

These principles aren't rocket science. They are based upon an understanding of how women live and eat. They also incorporate what we have learned from the latest diet trends and the best of evidence-based medicine in nutrition science. A lot of them are common sense. But so many women have been so confused by a smokescreen

---

**The Body-*for*-LIFE for Women Eating Method is about . . .**

• The quality of food: Are you eating Smart Foods 80 percent of the time?

• The quantity of food: Are you paying attention to portion sizes?

• The frequency of food: Are you eating small meals made up of Smart Proteins, Smart Carbs, and Smart Fats five or six times a day?

of conflicting nutrition information, so turned around by a never-ending parade of fads and gimmicks, that they may have forgotten how to eat like, well, a normal person. The way of eating presented here recalibrates your eating habits. And it's as simple to follow as it is effective.

1. **Create your meals with the "Body-*for*-LIFE Smart Foods Table."** You're a woman; there are enough complications in your life. I promise not to add to them. You don't have to obsess about calories, fat grams, or carb counts. You just need to know some key basics and then customize your own daily eating plan, using the "Smart Foods Table" on page 106. It tells you exactly what you can eat and in what portions and servings. It's like going into a clothing store. You know that designer clothes are a lot more expensive than ready-to-wear, so you check the label before you buy. Same here. A serving of starchy corn or potatoes is "more expensive" than a serving of nonstarchy carrots or broccoli.

2. **Go for quality: Eat Smart Foods 80 percent of the time.** I don't want you to get all perfectionistic on me. You know—I tell you what to do, you try to do it perfectly. *Fuhgeddaboudit!* All that's required is that you follow the Body-*for*-LIFE for Women Eating Method principles 80 percent of the time. You'll have days when you're 150 percent with the program, and others when you can't tie your shoes, let alone avoid Junk Carbs. Of course, if you're PMS-ed out of your brain, forgive yourself for indulging in a few select Junk-Food-ridden indiscretions.

The 80 percent rule gives you wiggle room when you need it. It reduces the chance that you'll engage in more self-hate and self-denigration when you can't pull off being "perfect." It's your colleague's birthday? For God's sake, have a slice of cake and take the time to *taste* it, and really savor the experience. It's your anniversary? Go out and enjoy that romantic dinner for two. By learning the fine art of regrouping, you'll know you can get right back in the saddle the next day. If you're not sure, before you eat that cake or that dinner, ask yourself: "Will eating this cause me to lose control and binge?" Be honest. If the answer is yes, pass it up. It's not worth going through the hell of another binge. If the answer is no, have one serving and enjoy it.

3. **Focus on quantity: Keep track of portions and servings.** Do you serve your partner that Mount St. Pasta and then eat the same, huge portion? No can do.

*(continued on page 100)*

## Find Your BMI

To use the table, find the appropriate height in the left-hand column. Move across to a given weight. The number at the top of the column (in the shaded bar) is the body mass index (BMI) at that height and weight. Pounds have been rounded off.

| BMI | 19 | 20 | 21 | 22 | 23 | 24 | 25 | 26 | 27 | 28 |
|---|---|---|---|---|---|---|---|---|---|---|
| Height (in) | Weight (lb) | | | | | | | | | |
| 58 | 91 | 96 | 100 | 105 | 110 | 115 | 119 | 124 | 129 | 134 |
| 59 | 94 | 99 | 104 | 109 | 114 | 119 | 124 | 128 | 133 | 138 |
| 60 | 97 | 102 | 107 | 112 | 118 | 123 | 128 | 133 | 138 | 143 |
| 61 | 100 | 106 | 111 | 116 | 122 | 127 | 132 | 137 | 143 | 148 |
| 62 | 104 | 109 | 115 | 120 | 126 | 131 | 136 | 142 | 147 | 153 |
| 63 | 107 | 113 | 118 | 124 | 130 | 135 | 141 | 146 | 152 | 158 |
| 64 | 110 | 116 | 122 | 128 | 134 | 140 | 145 | 151 | 157 | 163 |
| 65 | 114 | 120 | 126 | 132 | 138 | 144 | 150 | 156 | 162 | 168 |
| 66 | 118 | 124 | 130 | 136 | 142 | 148 | 155 | 161 | 167 | 173 |
| 67 | 121 | 127 | 134 | 140 | 146 | 153 | 159 | 166 | 172 | 178 |
| 68 | 125 | 131 | 138 | 144 | 151 | 158 | 164 | 171 | 177 | 184 |
| 69 | 128 | 135 | 142 | 149 | 155 | 162 | 169 | 176 | 182 | 189 |
| 70 | 132 | 139 | 146 | 153 | 160 | 167 | 174 | 181 | 188 | 195 |
| 71 | 136 | 143 | 150 | 157 | 165 | 172 | 179 | 186 | 193 | 200 |
| 72 | 140 | 147 | 154 | 162 | 169 | 177 | 184 | 191 | 199 | 206 |
| 73 | 144 | 151 | 159 | 166 | 174 | 182 | 189 | 197 | 204 | 212 |
| 74 | 148 | 155 | 163 | 171 | 179 | 186 | 194 | 202 | 210 | 218 |
| 75 | 152 | 160 | 168 | 176 | 184 | 192 | 200 | 208 | 216 | 224 |
| 76 | 156 | 164 | 172 | 180 | 189 | 197 | 205 | 213 | 221 | 230 |

| 29 | 30 | 31 | 32 | 33 | 34 | 35 | 36 | 37 | 38 | 39 | 40 |
|----|----|----|----|----|----|----|----|----|----|----|----|

**Weight (lb)**

| 29 | 30 | 31 | 32 | 33 | 34 | 35 | 36 | 37 | 38 | 39 | 40 |
|----|----|----|----|----|----|----|----|----|----|----|----|
| 138 | 143 | 148 | 153 | 158 | 162 | 167 | 172 | 177 | 181 | 186 | 191 |
| 143 | 148 | 153 | 158 | 163 | 168 | 173 | 178 | 183 | 188 | 193 | 198 |
| 148 | 153 | 158 | 163 | 168 | 174 | 179 | 184 | 189 | 194 | 199 | 204 |
| 153 | 158 | 164 | 169 | 174 | 180 | 185 | 190 | 195 | 201 | 206 | 211 |
| 158 | 164 | 169 | 175 | 180 | 186 | 191 | 196 | 202 | 207 | 213 | 218 |
| 163 | 169 | 175 | 180 | 186 | 191 | 197 | 203 | 208 | 214 | 220 | 225 |
| 169 | 174 | 180 | 186 | 192 | 197 | 204 | 209 | 215 | 221 | 227 | 232 |
| 174 | 180 | 186 | 192 | 198 | 204 | 210 | 216 | 222 | 228 | 234 | 240 |
| 179 | 186 | 192 | 198 | 204 | 210 | 216 | 223 | 229 | 235 | 241 | 247 |
| 185 | 191 | 198 | 204 | 211 | 217 | 223 | 230 | 236 | 242 | 249 | 255 |
| 190 | 197 | 204 | 210 | 216 | 223 | 230 | 236 | 243 | 249 | 256 | 262 |
| 196 | 203 | 210 | 216 | 223 | 230 | 236 | 243 | 250 | 257 | 263 | 270 |
| 202 | 209 | 216 | 222 | 229 | 236 | 243 | 250 | 257 | 264 | 271 | 278 |
| 208 | 215 | 222 | 229 | 236 | 243 | 250 | 257 | 265 | 272 | 279 | 286 |
| 213 | 221 | 228 | 235 | 242 | 250 | 258 | 265 | 272 | 279 | 287 | 294 |
| 219 | 227 | 235 | 242 | 250 | 257 | 265 | 272 | 280 | 288 | 295 | 302 |
| 225 | 233 | 241 | 249 | 256 | 264 | 272 | 280 | 287 | 295 | 303 | 311 |
| 232 | 240 | 248 | 256 | 264 | 272 | 279 | 287 | 295 | 303 | 311 | 319 |
| 238 | 246 | 254 | 263 | 271 | 279 | 287 | 295 | 304 | 312 | 320 | 328 |

You need to stick to woman food portions. Let him down the plate of man food. <u>You'll need to learn what a portion of food is</u> (could be half of what you're eating now) and take a long, hard look at the portion sizes you're eating at home and when you dine out. <u>Most of us are just plain eating too much.</u>

The cornerstone of the Body-*for*-LIFE for Women Eating Method is to keep track of portion sizes and eat the appropriate number of servings per day of any food, based on your body mass index (BMI), the body's ratio of weight to height. (To calculate your BMI, see "Find Your BMI" on page 98. Also, be sure to note the health implications of your current BMI on the chart "BMI and Your Health.")

Let's tackle portion sizes first. Use the chart below to help you gauge the most appropriate portion for each type of food.

| Food | Portion Size |
|---|---|
| Rice or pasta | Size of a lightbulb |
| Baked potato (5 oz) | Size of a computer mouse |
| Bagel (half) | Size of a hockey puck |
| Muffin | Size of a large egg |
| Meats | Size of your palm |
| Nuts | Size of a ping-pong ball |
| Butter | Size of the tip of your thumb |
| Cheese | Size of two dice |
| Raw vegetables | Size of your fist (1 cup) |
| Cooked vegetables | Size of a lightbulb (½ cup) |
| Fruit | Size of a tennis ball |

**BMI and Your Health**

Body mass index can be an early indicator of your risk of developing chronic conditions such as heart disease and diabetes. Toxic Fat around your middle escalates this risk even more. Check this chart to see where you stand now, and notice how your health prognosis will dramatically improve by removing excess weight and inches.

| BMI | Medical Definition | Disease Risk IF WAIST LESS THAN OR EQUAL TO 40 IN. (MEN) OR 35 IN. (WOMEN) | Disease Risk IF WAIST GREATER THAN 40 IN. (MEN) OR 35 IN. (WOMEN) |
|---|---|---|---|
| 18.5 or less | Underweight | — | N/A |
| 18.5–24.9 | Normal | — | N/A |
| 25.0–29.9 | Overweight | Increased | High |
| 30.0–34.9 | Obese | High | Very high |
| 35.0–39.9 | Obese | Very high | Very high |
| 40 or greater | Extremely obese | Extremely high | Extremely high |

Next, determine what is an appropriate number of Smart Food servings for your plate.

If you're of normal weight (BMI under 25):

• If you're active (doing about an hour of exercise a day), eat five servings of Smart Proteins and five servings of Smart Carbohydrates (of which at least two are fruit and the rest whole grain foods, including one starchy veggie, if you wish). In addition, enjoy unlimited amounts of nonstarchy vegetables a day (at least five servings) and two or three servings of Smart Fats, including olive or canola oil and nuts.

• If you're *not* active (averaging about 20 minutes or less of physical activity per day), reduce Smart Proteins to four, reduce Smart Fats to one or two servings, and keep everything else the same.

## Cut Calories without Counting Them

Foods contain calories. And it doesn't take a rocket scientist to calculate that a Krispy Kreme doesn't quite cut it, calorie-wise (not to mention nutrient-wise), with a bowl of freshly steamed veggies and brown rice. We also know that most women just plain eat too many calories relative to their physical activity level, age, and body composition. But if the last thing you want to do is count calories, try managing them with these three easy tricks.

**1. Go for high-volume foods.** Foods with a high energy density have lots of calories in one serving and tend to contain less water. Low-energy-density foods, on the other hand, contain fewer calories and more water—thus, they are high-volume foods. That's why you can eat two, three, or more servings of a high-volume food for the same calories of a minuscule serving of a high-energy-density food. We're talking volume, ladies: The bigger the food volume, the lower the energy density, the smaller the calorie count. A perfect example: raisins versus grapes. A 100-calorie serving of raisins fills ¼ cup. A 100-calorie serving of grapes fills almost 2 cups.

Instead of scarfing down a whole bowl of brown rice, which has a high energy density (more calories), opt for a bowl of vegetables combined with ½ cup of brown rice, which is much less energy dense (fewer calories). The vegetables and rice together will fill you up and satisfy you better than that bowl of rice alone (you don't get the surge in insulin levels, followed by plummeting blood sugar). A sliced apple with peanut butter has far less energy density than a bagel with cream cheese does.

**2. Practice portion control.** So many of my patients say, "But I'm eating healthy food and still can't remove the weight!" That's because they're eating too much healthy food. Pare down your portions! Most women can achieve excellent results simply by paying attention to their serving sizes every time they eat. This means you snackers and pickers out there, too. Bits of this and bites of that add up to portions. And at restaurants, when in doubt, halve the portion in front of you and pack it up or give the rest away.

**3. Read food labels.** Thirty grams of fat in 1 cup (½ pint) of Ben and Jerry's. Who knew? When you read food labels, you increase your awareness of calories, carbs, fats, and proteins—and head for Smart Foods with low energy density and high volume, which fill you up instead of out.

If you're overweight (BMI over 25):

• If you're active (doing about an hour of exercise a day), eat five servings of Smart Proteins and five servings of Smart Carbohydrates (of which at least two are fruit and the rest whole grain foods, including one starchy veggie if you wish). Enjoy unlimited amounts of nonstarchy vegetables a day (at least five servings) and two or three servings of Smart Fats, including olive or canola oil and nuts.

• If you're *not* active (averaging about 20 minutes or less of physical activity per day), eat five servings of Smart Proteins, reduce your Smart Carbs to four servings, reduce Smart Fats to one or two, and keep everything else the same, including unlimited amounts of nonstarchy vegetables (at least five servings a day).

(*Note*: Some women find it difficult to watch their weight without counting calories. If this sounds like you, see Appendix D, page 223, to figure out what works best for you.)

**4. Eat frequently: Choose Smart Foods every 2 to 4 hours, for a total of five or six meals a day.** A baby cries for food every 2 to 4 hours like clockwork. When men's stomachs rumble, they eat. (Maybe not the best food, but they eat.) Women? They ignore their rumbling stomachs for as long as possible, running around and taking care of everyone but themselves. That isn't going to fly on this program. You'll be working your muscles, and they'll need to be fed.

I want you to eat *at least* five times a day: breakfast, a midmorning snack, lunch, a midafternoon snack, and dinner. You can also have an after-dinner snack, if you need one. Try not to eat 1 to 2 hours before you turn in, though: Because most women are not as active at night as they are during the day, you probably won't burn off those calories. I have a saying: "Eat after 8, pack on the weight." Remember my 80 percent rule—it's okay to strive to hit this goal 80 percent of the time, so there's wiggle room. When life hits the fan, I don't expect you to not eat a nutritious dinner just because it's 9:00 P.M.!

Eating smaller meals, more often, will supply your growing muscles with a steady supply of fuel. Second, fueling like this will keep your metabolism revving so you'll burn more calories. (Frequent feedings reassure your body that there's no impending famine, so it's willing to part with fat. Skipping meals or going on a starvation diet counts as "famine.") Third, you prevent the dips in blood sugar that can leave you tired and irritable and craving empty calories like sweets and salty snacks. And finally, eating every 2 to 4 hours keeps you satisfied so that you never approach the next meal overly hungry. Stay satisfied, and you'll avoid overcompensating with extra calories. Whether you tend to skip meals, eat compulsively, or stick to three squares a day, you'll be pleasantly surprised by how good you feel—and by how the fat starts melting away.

**5. Plan your meals in advance and record what you eat.** I teach my patients, "If you fail to plan, you plan to fail." True in business, and true when you're exchanging unhealthy eating habits for new, healthy ones. Remember—you're doing this program for you, so you can take 10 minutes to pack your lunch or prepare take-along healthy snacks. Use the Daily Progress Report on page 217 to plan your meals in advance and record what you eat. The Daily Progress Report is a cinch to use. It even helps you keep track of your water intake. And filling out your daily journal ensures that you won't "forget" those M&M's you snitched from a colleague's desk, or the french fries you stole off your child's plate. Research shows that women who keep food journals are the most successful at weight loss because they learn to be accountable. A food journal is like a checkbook: You've got to know what's in there, or there's hell to pay. (See page 120 for a sample food journal page.)

**6. Eat two or three servings of calcium-rich foods a day.** You know that calcium helps prevent osteoporosis (see "Choose a Female-Friendly Multi" on page 116). But did you know it can help you remove weight? Research now shows how this mineral can influence fat cells to release their fat fuel more efficiently, especially if your calcium is from fat-free or low-fat dairy products. This mineral packs even more female-friendly benefits, including easing PMS and protecting against colon and breast cancers. You can get your calcium from low-fat or fat-free dairy products or from calcium-rich foods other than dairy. Nondairy sources of calcium, like broccoli or calcium-fortified OJ, are every bit as good as the kind that comes from Bessie.

**7. Drink 11 or 12 (8-ounce) glasses of water a day.** Water truly is the elixir of life—your Body-*for*-LIFE! It boosts your energy and detoxifies the body, and on this program, you gotta drink up. The Institute of Medicine of the National Academies recently set dietary intake levels for water. Its report said that women who appear to be adequately hydrated consume about 91 ounces of total water a day (about 11 glasses) from everything they eat and drink. My patients and colleagues are used to seeing me hauling around my water bottle. I also like some of the flavored waters—they set me back only 10 calories, and they taste terrific.

Drinking enough water also discourages water weight, the bane of many a puffy woman. (When your body doesn't get enough fluids, your kidneys hold on to the water they have.) Plus, water makes your stomach feel fuller, which will curb your appetite. A University of Washington study found that drinking one glass of water shut down appetite in 100 percent of subjects.

And finally, here's some news you can use. Betcha didn't know that drinking ice water encourages weight removal. Seriously. The energy required to raise the temperature of ice water to the body's core temperature can amount to a removal of several pounds of weight by the end of a year.

**8. Take Mini Chills when you need to.** Sometimes only chocolate will do. Rest assured, the Body-*for*-LIFE for Women Eating Method does not doom you to a life without it. Read on to learn more about the Mini Chill. I guarantee, you'll love it.

## SO WHAT CAN YOU EAT?

Take a look at the Smart Foods in the table on page 106. You'll see four main groups: Smart Proteins, Smart Carbs, Smart Fats, and Smart Snacks. (I've added a fifth group—Junk Foods—to show you what *not* to eat.) For each main meal, simply choose one food from each of groups A and B, and a half serving of C, in any combination, and add *at least* one nonstarchy veggie from group B to at least two of your meals. Remember, you can also add unlimited quantities of nonstarchy vegetables to any meal. For example, for breakfast you might opt for an egg-white veggie omelet (group A and group B, cooked in group C) and a slice of whole wheat toast (group B). For dinner, you might have swordfish (group A) with a sweet potato (starchy, group B), rounded out with green beans and zucchini (both nonstarchy group B). When you eat a snack (between breakfast and lunch, for example), use the same principles; you can also choose from group D, Smart Snacks.

*(continued on page 108)*

## Body-*for*-LIFE Smart Foods Table

For the next 12 weeks, as you follow the Body-*for*-LIFE for Women Eating Method, you'll be creating your meals and snacks from the table of yummy foods below (and in the indicated serving sizes). Aim for three meals and at least two snacks per day, about 2 to 4 hours apart (with 3 being

### GROUP A—SMART PROTEINS

| Eggs, Cheese, and Reduced-Fat Dairy | Fish (4 oz) | Soy Foods/Meat Substitutes |
|---|---|---|
| Cheese, light or fat-free, 2 oz | Catfish | Soy chicken patty, 1 |
| Low-fat yogurt, 8 oz | Haddock | Soy burger, 1 |
| Whole egg, 1 | Salmon | Soy hot dog, 1 |
| Egg whites, 3 or 4 | Shellfish (shrimp, crab, lobster) | Soy cheese, 2 oz |
| Egg substitutes, 1/3–1/2 cup | Tuna | Soy milk, 8 oz |
| Low-fat cottage cheese, 1/2 cup | **Meat or Poultry (3–4 oz)** | Soy nuts, 1/4–1/3 cup |
| Low-fat (1%) or fat-free milk, 8 oz | Skinless chicken or turkey | Tofu, 4 oz |
| Fat-free ricotta cheese, 1/3 cup | Lean beef or pork | |
| | Lean deli meat | |

### GROUP B—SMART CARBOHYDRATES

| Vegetables (1/2 cup cooked or 1 cup raw) | | |
|---|---|---|
| Artichoke | Lettuce | Citrus fruits (orange, grapefruit) |
| Asparagus | Mushrooms | Dried fruit, 1/4 cup |
| Beans | Onions | Watermelon, cantaloupe |
| Broccoli | Peas (starchy) | |
| Brussels sprouts | Potato, sweet (starchy) | **Whole grains (limit to 2 per day)** |
| Cabbage | Pumpkin | Whole grain bread, 1 slice |
| Carrots | Spinach | Whole wheat bagel, pita or wrap, 1/2 |
| Cauliflower | Squash | |
| Celery | Tomato | Steamed brown rice, 1/2 cup cooked |
| Corn (starchy) | Zucchini | Steamed wild rice, 1/2 cup cooked |
| Cucumber | **Fruits (1 whole fruit or 1 cup berries or melon chunks)** | Whole grain pasta, 1/2 cup cooked |
| Green beans | Apple | Oatmeal, 1/2 cup cooked |
| Green peppers | Berries (strawberries, blueberries) | Barley, 1/2 cup cooked |

optimal). To make a meal, choose a portion of protein from group A and carbohydrates from group B, and add an extra serving of nonstarchy vegetables from group B to at least two of your daily meals. Season your meals with a half serving of nuts or oils from group C, Smart Fats.

**GROUP C—SMART FATS**

Avocado, ¼

Nuts: 15 almonds, 20 peanuts, 12 walnut halves (also can count as Smart Proteins)

Olive oil, 1 tablespoon

Canola oil, 1 tablespoon

Safflower oil, 1 tablespoon

**GROUP D—SMART SNACKS**

½ portion of any Smart Protein with ½ portion of any Smart Carb

1 tablespoon nut butter on celery or on 1 sliced apple

Any nonstarchy veggie, anytime

½ portion of nuts mixed with ½ portion of dried fruit

½ whole wheat bagel and hummus

**GROUP E—JUNK FOODS (ELIMINATE OR EAT SPARINGLY)**

Processed foods: White sugar, white pasta, cookies, chips, pastries, candy bars, soda

Processed meats: Bologna, hot dogs, sausage

Full-fat red meat, dairy, and cheese (high in saturated fat)

Any food with trans fats

Because you'll be enjoying Smart Foods for the next 12 weeks—and, for that matter, the rest of your life—let's take a closer look at what makes them nutritional all-stars, and learn more about each category.

## SMART PROTEINS

Research has shown that it is protein, not fat or carbs, that is most satisfying. One serving (like a low-fat string cheese, yogurt, cottage cheese, or a handful of nuts) nips carb cravings in the bud and keeps you going for 2 or 3 hours. Yet women typically

---

### I Follow Mouth Principles, Too

I'm what you call a fish vegetarian—I eat fish, dairy, and eggs. But except for the poultry and red meat thing, my fish vegetarianism is pretty similar to the Body-*for*-LIFE for Women Eating Method. For example, both are composed of Smart Foods, like fruits, veggies, whole grains, soy, and fish, and both include the Smart Proteins, Smart Carbs, and Smart Fats that a woman's body needs.

My fish vegetarianism suits me. You like red meat? Rock on. Just make sure you get the leanest cuts and eat it in appropriate serving sizes. I've noticed, however, that more and more women are becoming vegetarians, or at least part-time vegetarians. That's not surprising—according to one survey, twice as many women as men in this country are vegetarians. (Men love slabs of beef? I'm shocked.) In addition, women can get all the female-friendly nutrients they need from a vegetarian diet—even the U.S. Dietary Guidelines say so. The two most common vegetarian diets are lacto-ovo (includes eggs and milk products, but not meat) and vegan (no animal products).

If you're interested in learning more about vegetarianism, I encourage you to check out the Vegetarian Diet Pyramid, developed in 1998 by nutrition scientists and medical specialists from Cornell University, the Harvard School of Public Health, and the Oldways Preservation and Exchange Trust in Cambridge, Massachusetts. To see the Pyramid, log on to www.oldwayspt.org/pyramids/veg/p_veg.html.

Finally, I make sure to take my vitamins every day. These include a multivitamin, as well as two 1,000-milligram omega-3 fish oil supplements, 1,500 milligrams of calcium, and my 100 milligrams of $CoQ_{10}$.

bypass the protein and flock to what I call grab-and-go carbs, like bagels, cookies, and doughnuts. Grab-and-go carbs—synonymous with Junk Carbs—don't satisfy your hunger. In fact, they tend to drive up your craving for more Junk Carbs. The Smart Proteins below will leave you full and happy—but not stuffed.

### Chicken and Turkey

Cooked without fat and eaten without the skin, chicken and turkey are low in fat, high in protein, relatively inexpensive, and incredibly versatile. Ground poultry makes delicious meat loaf, tacos, or burgers. But when you shop at the meat counter, specify that you want ground breast meat. Most ground poultry contains dark meat, which raises its fat and calorie content. Boneless, skinless breasts work well with quick, low-fat cooking methods like stir-frying, grilling, and microwaving. Experiment with rubs and herb blends to add flavor.

Quick tip: No time to cook? Many supermarkets carry precooked boneless chicken strips and breasts, whole roasted chickens, and prepackaged sliced chicken breasts.

### Fish and Shellfish

Fish is an excellent source of lean protein, which you need for building firm, shapely muscle. But it also helps to protect a muscle you can't see: the heart muscle.

After analyzing 16 years of data involving almost 85,000 women, researchers in the prestigious Nurses' Health Study found that women who ate fish just once a week have a heart attack risk that is 29 percent lower than those who eat it less than once a month. And women who eat it five times a week have nearly half the risk of dying of a heart attack. Researchers credit omega-3 fatty acids. (*Note:* The FDA advises women who are pregnant or who may become pregnant, nursing mothers, and young children to limit their intake of certain fish—tuna, swordfish, tilefish, king mackerel, and shark. These fish contain high levels of mercury, a toxic metal, which may cause neurological problems in a child or an unborn fetus.) Also, it's best to purchase wild salmon and not farmed salmon, which may contain high levels of toxic PCBs and dioxin.

Quick tip: The fish that pack the most omega-3s are sardines, mackerel, herring, whitefish, lake trout, chub, anchovy, wild chinook salmon, albacore tuna, bluefish, and halibut. Runners-up: wild coho salmon, rainbow trout, and cod.

*(continued on page 112)*

## A Look at Energy Bars

Clearly, in the best of all worlds, we're always striving to eat fresh whole foods. But what do you do when you're stuck in a car, plane, or train with no access to smart choices? Well, you go to Plan B—and B is for *bars*. The best include a balance of fat (2 to 7 grams of fat, 0 to

| Brand | Calories | Fat Calories | Fat (g) |
|---|---|---|---|
| Zone Perfect | 200–210 | 60 | 6–7 |
| Luna | 170–180 | 35–40 | 4–4.5 |
| Odwalla | 220–260 | 20–70 | 2.5–7 |
| Odwalla Super Protein | 240 | 45 | 5 |
| Kashi Go Lean | 280–290 | 45–50 | 5–6 |
| Kashi Go Lean Crunchy | 140–170 | 25–35 | 3–4 |
| Dr. Soy | 170–185 | 25–35 | 2.5–4 |
| Genisoy | 220–260 | 40–50 | 3.5–6 |
| EAS Myoplex | 270 | 25 | 3 |
| Revival | 250 | 80 | 9 |
| Hi-Lo Crisp Bar | 110 | 30 | 3 |
| Balance | 200–210 | 50–70 | 6–7 |
| Power Bar—Performance | 230–240 | 20–30 | 2–3.5 |
| Power Bar—Protein Plus | 270–290 | 45–50 | 5 |
| Power Bar—Harvest | 240–260 | 35–45 | 4–5 |
| Power Bar—Pria | 110 | 25 | 3 |
| Body-*for*-LIFE | 200–210 | 60–70 | 7 |
| SlimFast Optima | 220 | 45–50 | 5–6 |

4 grams of saturated fat), protein (10 to 20 grams), and carbohydrates (10 to 30 grams). They fit into a purse or a briefcase and can be a lifesaver when you're hungry and there's no other recourse. Best of all, you never have to get bored, because there's a wide range available. Here's a look at some of the more popular brands.

| Saturated Fat (g) | Sodium (mg) | Carbs (g) | Fiber (g) | Protein (g) |
|---|---|---|---|---|
| 3.5–4 | 320–340 | 21–24 | >1–2 | 14–16 |
| 3–3.5 | 50–135 | 26 | 3 | 10 |
| 0.5–2.5 | 30–180 | 38–47 | 3–5 | 4–8 |
| 1 | 190 | 31 | 3 | 16 |
| 3–4.5 | 140–280 | 45–50 | 6 | 13 |
| 1.5–2 | 150–220 | 26–32 | 5 | 8–9 |
| 2–3 | 105–190 | 26–28 | >1–1 | 11–12 |
| 2.5–3.5 | 130–300 | 18–34 | 1–3 | 14–15 |
| 1 | 330–350 | 23 | 3 | 42 |
| 4 | 250 | 33 | 4 | 19 |
| 0.5 | 180 | 14 | 1 | 8 |
| 1–4 | 75–230 | 21–24 | >1–3 | 14–15 |
| 0.5 | 90–120 | 45 | 2–3 | 9–10 |
| 2.5–3.5 | 140–220 | 36–38 | 1–2 | 24 |
| 0.5–2 | 80–125 | 45 | 2–4 | 7 |
| 2–2.5 | 79–90 | 16–17 | 0 | 5 |
| 3.5–4 | 160–270 | 21–22 | >1–1 | 15 |
| 3 | 75–250 | 33–35 | 2–3 | 8 |

**Low-Fat or Fat-Free Cottage Cheese, Ricotta Cheese, and Sliceable Cheeses**

Cottage cheese is high in protein and low in fat, and it's a good source of glutamine, an amino acid that helps support muscle metabolism. It's also a complete protein, which means it contains all the amino acids necessary to build new muscle. But this incredibly portable, versatile food also does a woman's bones good: Just ½ cup contains 69 milligrams of calcium, which helps ward off osteoporosis. Look for no-added-salt versions. Other good-for-you cheeses are fat-free ricotta cheese, which contains five times as much calcium as cottage cheese, and light or fat-free solid cheeses, such as American, Cheddar, and mozzarella.

**Quick tip:** For a yummy dessert, mix low-fat cottage cheese or low-fat ricotta cheese in a blender with one packet of Splenda (sucralose) and a handful of berries.

**Eggs and Egg Substitutes**

Whole eggs contain a variety of important nutrients and are an excellent source of protein, so I think it's fine to enjoy one egg a day. And the American Heart Association agrees. But egg whites are a nutritional bargain. Packed with protein, low in calories, and containing zero cholesterol and fat, egg whites cook up into delicious, fluffy scrambled eggs and omelets.

**Quick tip:** If you'd rather not use egg whites, try egg substitutes, such as Egg Beaters. Unlike whole eggs, these products have been pasteurized, which eliminates the risk of salmonella poisoning. That means you can pour 'em directly into the blender when you make a protein smoothie.

**Very Lean Red Meat or Deli Meat**

To many women, eating meat is a guilty pleasure—too much fat, too many calories, too much cholesterol. Right? Wrong. The leanest cuts of meat are excellent sources of protein and are low in fat. Plus, they're a good source of the trace mineral zinc, a nutrient that the average woman needs and often doesn't get enough of in her diet. Zinc boosts immunity and may even keep bones thick and strong. Meats are also an important source of iron.

**Quick tip:** When possible, choose "select," the leanest grade of beef. Whatever the grade, you'll get the least fat from beef cuts that include "round" in the name. Best bets: The leanest cuts of beef include eye round, top round, and top sirloin.

**Soy Foods (Tofu, Soy Milk/Yogurt, Soy Nuts, Meat Analogs)**

These foods are made from soybeans and are excellent sources of low-fat, high-fiber, nutrient-dense protein. Quality-wise, soy protein is equal to animal protein but minus the cholesterol. Soy is also rich in phytoestrogens—substances in plants that have a weak estrogen effect when eaten. Phytoestrogens are a good thing for women in any Milestone: They may reduce the risk of uterine, breast, and colon cancers, help prevent heart disease and osteoporosis, and help ease hot flashes, night sweats, and other symptoms of perimenopause.

**Quick tip:** Soy analogs—that's soy burgers, soy hot dogs, or soy chicken patties—are actually quite tasty. No kidding! Plop 'em into a whole grain pita for a perfect balance of protein and carbs. Another tasty soy treat is edamame (eh-dah-MAH-meh), or fresh soybeans. Along with soy nuts, edamame makes a quick, tasty snack and is an excellent source of low-fat lean protein, fiber, iron, and calcium. You can find preshelled edamame in the frozen food section at health food stores.

## SMART CARBS

Your body will become leaner, fitter, and healthier with a diet that balances protein and carbohydrates. You can have as many nonstarchy veggies as you want—bring 'em on! Learn to grill and roast veggies to bring out their flavor.

You can also have at least two daily servings of fruit—yes, *fruit.* No matter what the low-carb gurus say, an orange or an apple here, ½ cup of berries there, won't cause weight gain. Fruit is wonderfully healthy, and its sugar (fructose) doesn't trigger the same roaring appetite for Junk Carbs that refined sugar does.

I recommend two or three servings max of whole grains per day, unless you're getting substantially more than the recommended physical activity in the Body-*for*-LIFE for Women Training Method. This is especially true if you're over the age of 40, when you have to be more aware of calorie-dense foods like whole grains and the physical activity price you have to pay to work 'em off. I recommend that you have your last serving no later than your midafternoon snack, and make dinner one serving of Smart Protein, lots of nonstarchy veggies, and maybe a serving of fruit as well.

I also suggest that you limit or eliminate white potatoes, pasta made with white flour, and bread (and even limit whole grain bread). These carbs are stripped of their valuable nutrients and raise hell with your insulin levels. When it comes to the "white" or processed carbs, I say, "If it's white, it's not right." If you must, have one small potato (it should fit in the palm of your hand), one serving of whole wheat pasta (½ cup), or one slice of 100 percent whole grain bread (or one small whole wheat pita or wrap, if you prefer). More often, go for the Smart Carbs below.

### Beans

Packed with fiber, vitamins, minerals, and phytochemicals, beans are awesomely nutritious. The canned ones are just as healthy as the dried kind, once you rinse them in water to get rid of the sodium-filled juice. Their fiber helps you feel fuller longer, and, like most carbohydrates from vegetables, beans generally have only a small effect on blood sugar and insulin.

Quick tip: Ladle some chickpeas from the salad bar onto your lunchtime salad; get them in a cup of soup at a diner; make your five-alarm chili with beans instead of beef.

### Berries

Berries are packed with nutritional riches. They contain phytonutrients, the pigments that give fruits their crayon-bright colors. For instance, blueberries contain tannins, compounds that help fight urinary tract infections, and strawberries contain ellagic acid (a powerful anticancer agent), as well as antioxidants and fiber. Berries are also quite low in carbohydrates; ½ cup of whole strawberries contains just 5 grams of carbohydrates, and 3 of those are fiber!

Quick tip: Before you buy berries, give the carton a quick once-over. If it's stained with juice, the berries at the bottom are probably not in good shape; choose another. Store berries uncovered in the refrigerator, and eat them as soon as possible: They don't keep for long. Or freeze some to enjoy later; freezing preserves important nutrients, such as vitamin C.

### Low-Fat Plain Yogurt

With 300 to 400 milligrams of calcium per cup, low-fat plain yogurt is one of the best sources of bone-saving calcium you can get. It also contains vitamin D, which your body needs for absorbing calcium. Try mixing fat-free yogurt and cottage cheese (sweetened with a little Splenda and sprinkled with cinnamon, if you like) for a quick, easy morning or evening meal. Frozen yogurt is too high in sugar to make the "authorized" list.

**Quick tip:** To make a quick vegetable dip, put yogurt in a sieve lined with a coffee filter and refrigerate for 3 or more hours. Then blend this yogurt "cheese" with chopped garlic, salt, pepper, and your favorite seasonings.

### Oatmeal, Brown Rice, and Barley

These whole grains are outstanding sources of complex carbohydrates, your body's preferred fuel. They're called "whole" grains because they've retained the bran and germ, which contain as much as 80 percent of their vitamins, minerals, and fiber and up to 50 percent of their protein. They are also rich in phytonutrients, plant-derived compounds that act as disease repellents. By contrast, white bread, white rice, and white pasta are refined grains, stripped of their nutritious outer layers.

Unless you work out after dinner, you're probably not burning a whole lot of calories after 5:00 P.M. So eat whole grains and other Smart Carb choices earlier in the day, when you can burn them off. Remember, the correct portion is one you can fit in the palm of your hand, or about the size of half a tennis ball. Other good-for-you grains include whole wheat couscous, quinoa, wheat berries, bulgur, hot and cold cereals made with whole grains like oatmeal, and wild rice.

**Quick tip:** Barley isn't just for soups. Try it for breakfast—it's delicious mixed with a little Splenda and cinnamon, or a dollop of low-fat fruit yogurt. Opt for hulled barley, the most nutritious type. You'll find it in health food stores.

### Sweet Potatoes

Believe it or not, sweet potatoes are not higher in calories than a regular spud. But they are stuffed with vitamin C, fiber, and beta-carotene, which help fight heart disease and cancer. Prepare them just as you would a regular potato—baked, boiled, or microwaved. You can even slice 'em thin, throw 'em in the oven on a pan, and bake your own "chips." But choose smaller sweet potatoes—the size of your clenched fist—or eat half and save the rest.

**Quick tip:** Try sprinkling a sweet potato with a dash of cinnamon. Delicious!

## SMART FATS

If the low-carb fad has shown anything, it's that you can remove weight while eating fat. Of course, you have to choose the right fats. And be mindful of portion size, because

*(continued on page 121)*

## Choose a Female-Friendly Multi

Here's a cheat sheet to the vitamins and minerals the female body needs for peak health. You can get many of them by following the Body-*for*-LIFE for Women Eating Method. I also recommend taking a daily multivitamin/mineral supplement. Stick to a well-known brand (Centrum and Theragram are two examples) that contains 100 percent of the Daily Value (DV) of the essential

### FAT-SOLUBLE VITAMINS

| Vitamin | Best Sources |
| --- | --- |
| Vitamin A | Plant sources: dark-colored fruits and leafy vegetables (carrots, winter squash, spinach), which the body converts to vitamin A; animal sources: low-fat or fat-free milk, eggs, low-fat or fat-free cheese, chicken |
| Vitamin D | Sunlight, fatty fish such as salmon or fish oils, egg yolks, low-fat or fat-free milk (dairy or soy), fortified orange juice, cereals enriched with vitamin D |
| Vitamin E | Vegetable oils, nuts, seeds, wheat germ, whole grains |

### WATER-SOLUBLE VITAMINS

| Vitamin | Best Sources |
| --- | --- |
| Vitamin C | Citrus fruits, tomatoes, green peppers, cabbage, green vegetables, mangoes, strawberries, cantaloupe, broccoli, cranberry juice |
| Vitamin $B_1$ (thiamin) | Whole grains, pork, sunflower seeds, beans, seafood |
| Vitamin $B_2$ (riboflavin) | Lean meats, fish, almonds, whole grains, low-fat or fat-free dairy products, dark green leafy vegetables, enriched breads, cereals, pasta (opt for whole grain) |
| Vitamin $B_3$ (niacin) | Whole grains, low-fat or fat-free dairy products, lean meats, poultry, fish, nuts, broccoli, peas, beans, brewer's yeast |

vitamins and minerals below. If you're over 50, opt for a "seniors" formula that contains extra vitamin D, vitamin B$_6$, vitamin B$_{12}$, and calcium. Unless you're still menstruating, forget the iron.

By the way, you won't find a multi with 100 percent of the DV of calcium. You can't absorb your entire quota of calcium all at once, and besides, that amount would turn your multi into a horse pill!

| Health/Wellness Benefits | Recommended Daily Dose |
|---|---|
| Antioxidant; necessary for good vision, healthy skin and mucous membranes, and overall growth and development | 4,000 IU* |
| Essential for bone and teeth formation; helps calcium and phosphorus get into bones; prevents osteoporosis; boosts immune function | Under 50 years old: 200–400 IU; over 50 years old: 400–800 IU |
| Protective antioxidant; boosts immune system; helps form blood cells and nerve tissue; may help prevent heart disease, cataracts, and cancer | 100–400 IU |

| Health/Wellness Benefits | Recommended Daily Dose |
|---|---|
| Protective antioxidant; immune booster—necessary for healthy gums, bones, teeth and skin, and blood vessels; helps in wound healing; may prevent cataracts; helps body absorb iron | 200–500 mg |
| Energy production from carbohydrates; forms red blood cells; maintains skeletal muscle | 1.1 mg |
| Helps in energy production; maintains healthy eyes, skin, nerves | 1.1 mg |
| Helps in energy production; maintains healthy brain function, proper blood circulation, and healthy skin | 14 mg |

*Taking more than 100 percent of the DV may cause bone fractures in postmenopausal women and is linked to birth defects and liver toxicity. Select a multi that has part or all of its vitamin A as beta-carotene; it's safer.*

(continued)

## Choose a Female-Friendly Multi—cont.

**WATER-SOLUBLE VITAMINS—CONT.**

| Vitamin | Best Sources |
|---|---|
| Vitamin $B_6$ | Chicken, fish, pork, lamb, milk, eggs, unmilled (brown) rice, whole grains, soybeans, potatoes, beans, nuts, seeds, and dark green leafy vegetables. (In the U.S., bread and other products made from refined grains are fortified with vitamin $B_6$.) |
| Vitamin $B_{12}$ | Low-fat or fat-free dairy products, eggs, lean meats, poultry, fish, fortified soy milk |
| Folic Acid | Dark green leafy vegetables, citrus fruits, beans and peas, wheat germ, whole/enriched grain products, mushrooms |
| Calcium | Low-fat or fat-free dairy products, canned salmon and sardines, sardines with bones, wild salmon, dark green leafy vegetables, tofu, fortified soy or rice milk, fortified orange juice |
| Iron | Lean meats, poultry, fish, dried beans, nuts, dried fruits (such as prunes and raisins), molasses, dark leafy green vegetables, cocoa, egg yolks, whole grains |
| Magnesium | Dark green leafy vegetables, nuts, figs, whole grains, dried peas and beans, low-fat or fat-free dairy products, fish, lean meats, poultry |
| Zinc | Red meats, poultry, oysters, eggs, legumes, nuts, low-fat or fat-free milk or yogurt, whole grain cereals, sesame and pumpkin seeds |

| Health/Wellness Benefits | Recommended Daily Dose |
|---|---|
| A component of enzymes that metabolize proteins and fats; essential for getting energy and nutrients from food; stored extensively in muscle tissue, thus available during intense physical activity; plays an important role in removing excess homocysteine from the blood, a substance thought to be responsible for a significant percentage of heart disease | 1.6 mg |
| Helps convert carbohydrates into energy; maintains red blood cells, nervous system; helps keep homocysteine levels low, which is important for heart health | 2.4 mcg |
| Protects newborns from congenital birth defects; needed for healthy red blood cells; prevents heart disease by lowering homocysteine levels; lowers risk of colon cancer | 400 mcg |
| Necessary for maintaining healthy bones, teeth, bone strength, muscle function; helps prevent osteoporosis; may reduce blood pressure | 1,200 mg† |
| Helps in energy production; essential for red blood cells that transfer oxygen throughout the body‡ | Before menopause: 18 mg; after menopause: 8 mg |
| Antioxidant; immune booster; essential for healthy muscle and nerve function and bone formation; may help with PMS; may help prevent heart disease, diabetes, osteoporosis, hypertension, and migraines | Up to age 30: 310 mg; after age 30: 320 mg |
| Essential for wound healing, cell reproduction, normal growth and development, healthy skin, and resistance to infection | 8 mg (16 mg for vegans) |

†*Most women can't get this amount from food. I tell my patients to take calcium hydroxyapatite or calcium citrate supplements. (Avoid calcium carbonate supplements, which aren't absorbed as well and cause GI upset in many women.) Important: Choose a calcium supplement fortified with vitamin D, which helps the body absorb calcium.*

‡*Including a source of vitamin C, such as orange juice, increases absorption of iron.*

## Sample Eating Plan

| *Body-for-LIFE for Women* | *Mind-Mouth-Muscle Daily Journal: Mouth* |
|---|---|
| Date: December 10 | Day <u>15</u> of 84 |

| | |
|---|---|
| Total portions of Smart Protein:  6 | Total portions of Smart Protein:  6 |
| Total portions of Smart Carbs:  8 | Total portions of Smart Carbs:  8 |
| Total portions of Smart Fats:  2 | Total portions of Smart Fats:  2 |

| PLAN | ACTUAL |
|---|---|
| MEAL 1 ☑ A.M. ☐ P.M. — ½ cup cooked oatmeal with ½ scoop vanilla protein powder / ¾ cup skim or 1% milk, dairy or soy / ½ cup blueberries / 5–6 walnuts halves | MEAL 1 ☑ A.M. ☐ P.M. — ½ cup cooked oatmeal with ½ scoop vanilla protein powder / ¾ cup skim milk / ½ cup blueberries / 6 walnuts halves |
| MEAL 2 ☑ A.M. ☐ P.M. — small yogurt with ¼ cup fat-free cottage cheese / medium banana | MEAL 2 ☑ A.M. ☐ P.M. — small yogurt / medium banana |
| MEAL 3 ☐ A.M. ☑ P.M. — 4 cups salad greens / 4 oz tuna in foil pack / 4 tsp 50/50 olive oil and vinegar mix | MEAL 3 ☐ A.M. ☑ P.M. — 4 cups salad greens / 4 oz tuna in foil pack / 4 tsp 50/50 olive oil and vinegar mix |
| MEAL 4 ☐ A.M. ☑ P.M. — 2 light string cheese sticks / 1 medium apple | MEAL 4 ☐ A.M. ☑ P.M. — Nutrition Bar |
| MEAL 5 ☐ A.M. ☑ P.M. — 4 oz. cooked salmon / 4 spears asparagus / ½ cup cooked carrots / ½ cup red bell peppers | MEAL 5 ☐ A.M. ☑ P.M. — 4 oz. chicken breast / 4 spears asparagus / ½ cup cooked carrots / ½ cup tomatoes |
| MEAL 6 ☐ A.M. ☑ P.M. — 1 cup sugar-free pudding made with fat-free milk / 1 cup fresh fruit mix: melon, grapes, berries | MEAL 6 ☐ A.M. ☑ P.M. — 1 cup sugar-free pudding made with fat-free milk / 1 cup fresh fruit mix: melon, grapes, berries |

*Veggies* ☑ ☑ ☑ ☑

*Calcium-rich foods* ☑ ☑ ☑

*Water* ☑ ☑ ☑ ☑ ☑ ☑ ☑ ☑ ☑ ☑

*Mini Chill* ☐

HOW DID YOU DO?

<u>Didn't need the Mini Chill because the nutrition bar</u>

<u>was chocolate—yum!</u>

a mere tablespoon contains about 120 calories. There are two specific kinds of essential fats in the Body-*for*-LIFE for Women Eating Method: omega-6 fatty acids and omega-3 fatty acids. They're the only dietary fats a woman requires. These are found in olive, canola, and safflower oils, the oils found in fatty fish (wild salmon, tuna, halibut, to name three), in flax seeds or oil, and in dark green leafy vegetables, such as spinach. As long as you eat adequate amounts of the foods that contain them, you're golden.

Don't forget nuts, which are chock-full of heart-healthy mono- and polyunsaturated fats. The key is to remember the portion issue—nuts are high in calories. So you're talking 15 almonds, 20 peanuts, or 12 walnut halves.

**Quick tip:** To tell the good fats from the bad, give them the room temperature test. At room temperature, healthy fats, like safflower, canola, and olive oils, are liquid. Unhealthy ones, like butter, margarine, or shortening, are solid.

## CHILL OUT—HAVE SOME CHOCOLATE

A few pages back, I told you I wanted you to follow the Mouth way of eating 80 percent of the time. So what do you eat for the remaining 20 percent of the time?

Simple: something you want to eat. Maybe a cookie. A couple of bite-size chocolates. A half-cup of ice cream.

In other words, ladies, you take a Mini Chill—an opportunity during the week to splurge a bit. In my experience, women need these moments. Why? Because regardless of the Milestone we're in, our hormones play some serious havoc with our appetites, energy levels, and moods, and because we get hit with serious amounts of stress in the course of a day. So for crying out loud, if your period is due and you'd sell your mother for chocolate, go ahead and have a fun-size bar, and leave your mom alone!

Boy, do I love my Mini Chills. My favorite nonbingeable Junk Carb is a chocolate or almond biscotti with my mocha latte made with skim milk. When I'm perimenopausal out of my brain, I love to have one or two, hop in bed, watch reruns of *Sex and the City,* and turn in early. When I wake up, it's back to Smart Foods.

Sometimes, though, stress and hormones don't melt away in one day. Your job is to ride them out with the least self-destruction. If I'm still pooped out the next day, I stay focused on my eating and exercise but reserve the right to have another cookie if I feel like it. Feel free to do the same.

But be smart, now. Mini Chills aren't license for you to pig out or to eat foods you know will trigger a binge. Don't be surprised if, after a few weeks of indulging in Mini Chills, you have a week when you don't feel the need to indulge in even one. Or you find that a bowl of luscious fresh fruit with a little dollop of low-cal whipped topping is every bit as satisfying as candy or cookies. That is a sign that you're approaching balance in your eating. And that's what it's all about.

---

### Overview: The Body-*for*-LIFE for Women Eating Method

1. Create your meals with the Body-*for*-LIFE Smart Foods template. To make a meal, choose one food from each of groups A and B, and a half serving from C. Add an extra serving of non-starchy veggies to two or more of those meals. When you need a snack, use the same principles or choose from group D, Smart Snacks.

2. Go for quality: Eat Smart Foods 80 percent of the time. Trying to achieve perfection sets you up to fail. The 80 percent rule gives you wiggle room when you need it.

3. Focus on quantity: Keep track of portions and servings. Just as important, eat the appropriate number of servings per day of any food.

4. Heed frequency: Eat Smart Foods every 2 to 4 hours, for a total of five or six meals a day. That means at least five meals: breakfast, a midmorning snack, lunch, a midafternoon snack, and dinner. You can also have an after-dinner snack, if you need one.

5. Plan your meals in advance and record what you eat, using the Body-*for*-LIFE Daily Progress Report on page 217. The more you plan your meals, the more success you'll achieve.

6. Eat two or three servings of calcium-rich foods a day. You can get your calcium from low-fat or fat-free dairy products or from calcium-rich foods other than dairy.

7. Drink at least 11 or 12 glasses of water per day. Being adequately hydrated boosts your energy, helps your body eliminate toxins, and discourages water weight gain.

8. Take Mini Chills when you need to. Sometimes a woman's just gotta have it—chocolate, that is.

# Muscle: The Body-for-LIFE for Women Training Method

## Part 5

*"We are what we repeatedly do. Excellence then, is not an act, but a habit."*
—**Aristotle**

*"Those who think they have not time for bodily exercise will sooner or later have to find time for illness."*
—**Edward Stanley**

In 2001, 12 of my female patients and I dubbed ourselves the Peeke Performers, signed up for the 2001 New York City Marathon, and trained hard for 6 months. Then bright and early on a sunny November morning, we ran or walked the 26.2 miles through the five boroughs of New York City—6 weeks after the September 11 attacks. These women had weathered some heavy personal stuff—divorce, family crisis, big-time weight loss, serious illness—yet were up for one of the world's most daunting physical challenges.

In a way, my patient Betty founded the Peeke Performers. At the time of the 2001 marathon, she was undergoing treatment for recurring breast cancer; I was giving her nutritional and fitness advice. One day, I happened to mention that I'd entered the marathon. Betty said, "I want to do it with you." The word spread among my other patients, 11 more signed on for the marathon, and the Performers were born.

Betty crossed the finish line in 7 hours, 39 minutes, despite having undergone chemo just 3 days before. After that marathon—the fifth she has walked while raising funds for breast cancer research—Betty looked at me and said, "You know, I've always dreamed of climbing a mountain sometime before I die."

"No prob, Betty. This we can do," I said, and started shopping around for a mountain.

I found one in Colorado: Aspen's Green Mountain. The 3-day trip covered a lower-elevation mountain hike, a lake hike, and—the culmination of our trip—the climb to the summit of Green Mountain, elevation 13,700 feet.

Betty climbed. And climbed. The Performers all kept an eye on her progress, inspired by her every step.

We made it to the summit 4 hours after we'd set out. Once on the summit, we formed a circle. Holding hands, we gazed over the magnificent panorama, and one after another, each woman stepped into the middle of the circle and proclaimed her joy at having attained her goal. We picked mountain flowers, walked to the edge of the summit, and threw them into the air, letting them carry our joyful wishes over the mountaintops. It was magical.

The culmination of the hike was Betty tearfully and joyfully tossing her flowers into the summer winds with a wish to live her life to the fullest and savor each day as a precious gift.

As I write this, Betty is 63, still in remission, and as vibrant and energetic as always. And, in a way, she's still climbing. "I seized those precious moments and will hold them in my memory forever," she says. "Whenever I need to, I relive them. In my mind, I'm on the summit, gazing out over that glorious vista."

To hell with thin thighs. Screw the buns of steel. This is what fitness is all about. Betty knows it. The Peeke Performers know it. And whether or not you ever climb a mountain, so, someday, will you.

## YOU HAVE TO MOVE TO REMOVE WEIGHT

I see it over and over again. Desperate to remove weight, women reluctantly start a fitness program. In time, if they hang in there, a little miracle takes place. They discover that moving their bodies reshapes more than their hips or thighs or butt. It reshapes their lives. It empowers them to improve their lives in countless other ways.

So why don't women do it sooner?

As I write this, no more than 60 percent of American women get the daily recommended 30 minutes of physical activity. I'm not just talking about overweight women. I'm talking about *all* women. You may be thin, you may eat right, but if you're not active, you ain't as healthy as you think you are.

At least 25 percent of women are completely inactive—I'm talkin' one step over coma. This is not good. Studies conducted at prestigious research centers all over the nation have reached the same chilling conclusion: Overweight women, especially those carrying extra belly fat, are at increased risk of the metabolic syndrome—a combination of Toxic Fat, heart disease, diabetes, and cancer. *But it doesn't have to be this way.* Did you know that women who do 30 minutes of extra walking each day—at one time or accrued through the day—reduce their risk of breast cancer by 40 percent and their risks of heart disease and diabetes by half? That it takes only 60 to 90 minutes of exercise a week to significantly lower blood pressure? That moderate daily exercise works as well as antidepressants for women with mild depression and anxiety? Hello! Are you listening?

So quit growing roots in your chair at home or at work. To remove weight, you must move your weight. *Regularly.* When you do, wonderful things happen. You gain firm, sexy muscle. Preserve the density of your bones. Improve your mood. And most important, build the vital body that will keep you vertical and strong well into the last decades of your life.

The Muscle portion of the Body-*for*-LIFE for Women program will show you how to do both. The formula: a combination of cardio and resistance training, spiced with some flexibility exercises, and polished off with a bit more activity in everyday life. Whether your motivation is improved health or the desire to look great—or both!—this program can change your life.

One more thing. As you'll see later on, these first 12 weeks are the beginning of your journey. The Body-*for*-LIFE for Women Training Method is a program of transformation. Your exterior changes, yes, but so does your mind. When you make the investment in your most precious possession—yourself—I promise you that from here on in, life will only get better. You'll gain more than a fit body and mind. You'll also gain a deep sense of accomplishment and a heaping helping of self-respect.

## YOUR FITNESS NEEDS, MILESTONE BY MILESTONE

I've worked with thousands of women. Twenty-somethings to 50-plus career women. Anorexics and starvers to bingers and bulimics. Top athletes to women who were so obese that they could barely walk a block. For all of them, a customized fitness "prescription" became an essential part of their self-care.

Although women of every age reap tremendous physical and mental benefits from regular physical activity, age is a factor in how much and what kind of activity their bodies need in order to get fit, energetic, and strong. Here's a Milestone-by-Milestone description of a woman's physical activity needs.

### MILESTONE 1: MENSTRUATION TO FIRST PREGNANCY

Women in Milestone 1, with their surging estrogen and burgeoning breasts, hips, and thighs, typically have 21 to 32 percent body fat, well within a healthy range. They can keep this optimal level with regular physical activity. And because there's evidence that heart disease and diabetes can begin to develop in adolescence—even childhood—being active now, and staying active, can help protect them from heart disease, cancer, and diabetes down the road.

The benefits of fitness extend beyond physical health. Research shows that physical activity eases stress and depression in girls and that girls who play sports have a more positive body image and higher self-esteem than those who don't. For that matter, girls who are active in sports are less likely to contemplate suicide than girls who aren't; they tend to spend more time concentrating on their physical accomplishments and the fun of teamwork than obsessing about their weight. Another study shows that when preteens and teen girls get in just 30 to 40 minutes of exercise each day, they can lower by 30 percent their likelihood of developing breast cancer later in life.

### MILESTONE 2: THE REPRODUCTIVE YEARS

Women don't get fat from pregnancy. Their bodies simply are gaining the necessary reserves on hips and thighs to fuel the extra 500 calories a day required for breastfeeding. Women who enter pregnancy fit and stay physically active throughout the pregnancy are less likely to gain excess weight, and therefore, they have less to lose after they give birth. And being strong can definitely improve your endurance for the marathon of labor!

Of course, once the baby is born, a woman has to work to lose that excess fat, and the older you are when you deliver, the harder it is. Then, amid kids, career, the partner, and the whirlwind of everyday life, women in Milestone 2 face a most formidable challenge: to make physical activity a regular part of their high-stress lives. According to one study, being a mom cuts a woman's time for exercise by at least 20 percent. But putting in that sweat time is essential.

Regardless of whether a woman bears kids or not, beginning in her thirties, she normally loses 1 to 2 percent of her muscle per year, slowing her metabolism. She can even begin to lose bone. Regular physical activity revs up metabolism, preserves muscle, and slows bone loss.

It also safeguards her future health. Regular moderate-to-strenuous physical activity reduces a woman's risk for certain female cancers triggered by estrone, a type of estrogen that increases with higher-than-normal body fat and is associated with an increased risk of breast and uterine cancer. If you do regular physical activity from 1 to 3 hours a week from your teens to about age 40, you'll cut your risk of breast cancer by 20 to 30 percent. Four or more hours a week can reduce the risk almost 60 percent.

It's pretty simple: Move the weight, remove the weight, and reduce your risk.

## MILESTONE 3: PERIMENOPAUSE AND MENOPAUSE

Remember the way your body morphed at puberty? One day you were a beanpole, the next an hourglass. Well, once you hit 40, you're shape-shifting again. Although premenopausal women gain fat in the lower body to nourish children, women in Milestone 3, whose reproductive years are drawing to a close, gain it in their upper bodies. Think larger breasts, the emergence of back fat, weird little fat pouches near your armpits that hang over your bra, and the menopot. Hot flashes and other symptoms triggered by the swoops and dips of estrogen only add to the fun.

However! There's a huge difference between Milestone 3 women who are active and those who aren't. Women who stay fit through these years of hormonal fluctuations are less affected by the typical symptoms of menopause. They pack more lean muscle, have faster metabolisms, and can control their weight and body fat better. Physical activity also helps them control their blood sugar, blood pressure, and blood cholesterol, which become an issue for many women in this Milestone.

## MILESTONE 4: BEYOND MENOPAUSE

The goal of Milestone 4 women is to retain their functional independence and prevent disease. To do it, they need to pay special attention to achieving and maintaining adequate endurance, strength, and flexibility.

As a result of declining sex hormone levels, lack of physical activity, chronic stress, and overeating, women in this Milestone are at high risk for accumulating Toxic Fat. That's bad news, because apple-shaped women are at greater risk of heart disease than are pear-shaped women, who carry their weight on their hips, thighs, and bottoms. This extra weight can lead to chronic knee and back pain, which limit a woman's ability to get around.

Hormonal changes can also cause bone loss, raising a woman's risk of osteoporosis. In a recent study of nearly 90,000 women ages 50 to 64, almost one-third had bone density low enough to run an increased risk of fracture.

Happily, it doesn't take much physical activity to keep women in this Milestone fit and healthy. Weight training can build muscle, preserve bone, and improve strength, and simple walking can keep hearts beating strong. In one study, 73,743 women ages 50 to 79 were asked about their exercise habits, and those women who walked briskly or who engaged in more-intense exercise at least 2½ hours per week were *both* 30 percent less likely to develop cardiovascular disease than women who didn't do either.

I recommend that women in all Milestones—especially 3 and 4—seek out an experienced trainer who specializes in working with women 50 and over. Most midlife women have never lifted weights, and they need guidance to reduce the risk of training-related injuries. The price? Reasonable, and you need only a few sessions to learn proper form and technique, followed by perhaps monthly check-ins to make sure you're progressing well.

## THE MUSCLE FORMULA AT WORK:
## THE BODY-*FOR*-LIFE FOR WOMEN TRAINING METHOD

Every woman's fitness "prescription" is unique, based on her goals, habits, lifestyle, past athletic or physical fitness history, and overall health. That's why I designed the Body-*for*-LIFE for Women Training Method to be a bit like a buffet table. You take a little bit of this and a little bit of that, and you create your own made-to-order fitness program.

But simple as it is, the Body-*for*-LIFE for Women Training Method covers all five components of fitness: cardiovascular fitness (a.k.a. cardio), muscular strength, muscular endurance, flexibility, and balance. Each is vitally important to a woman's overall health and fitness, regardless of her age.

Here's the basic method. Just do me a favor. If you're over 40, have been sedentary for some time, or have a health condition, call your doctor and schedule a physical before you so much as pull on a gym sock.

**1. Perform some form of cardio 3 to 5 days a week for 30 minutes at a time.** Cardiovascular fitness—walking, running, swimming, rowing, Spinning, jumping rope— strengthens your heart and lungs, reduces body fat, and improves the body's ability to use glucose. It can also help reverse the resistance to insulin caused by Toxic Fat. (In one study, women who walked at least 3 hours a week had about a 40 percent lower risk of diabetes than did sedentary women.) Follow these guidelines, and you'll burn 200 to 500 calories per session, depending on your level of intensity (see "Go for the Burn" on page 132) and your level of fitness. You'll also increase your overall fitness level.

---

### The Body-*for*-LIFE for Women Training Method is about . . .

- The *quality* of movement: Are you working at full intensity?

- The *quantity* of movement: Are you accruing at least 30 minutes of cardio per workout and at least 30 minutes of resistance training per workout?

- The *frequency* of movement: Are you doing cardio at least three to five times a week and resistance training two or three times a week? Are you also moving more during the day?

### Walk It Off!

You know what a pedometer is—a device the size of a pager that records the number of steps you take. What you might not know is that folks who use pedometers tend to stay with their exercise program longer. What's more, in a study reported in the *Journal of the American Medical Association,* participants in a healthy lifestyle program who wore pedometers increased their activity levels by about 30 minutes, 5 days per week, and lost weight—doing nothing but inserting short "activity bursts" into their days!

I heartily recommend wearing a pedometer. Not only is it a simple way to monitor your progress, it also keeps you mindful of the importance of movement. Here's how to get the most from it.

Wear a pedometer for at least 3 days, from the time you get out of bed until you go to sleep at night. Do what you normally do. Try to measure at least one weekend day, because activity levels vary from weekdays. Calculate your baseline by averaging your step counts for the 3 days. Follow the chart below. Take as much time as you need to work up to your goal. Remember, every extra step counts!

| If Your Baseline Is . . . | Your Goal Is . . . | How to Reach |
|---|---|---|
| Less than 2,500 steps | 5,000 steps | Add 250 steps per day |
| 2,501–5,000 steps | 7,500 steps | Add 300 steps per day |
| 5,001–7,500 steps | 10,000 steps | Add 400 steps per day |
| 7,501–10,000 steps | 12,000 steps | Add 500 steps per day |
| 10,001–12,500 steps | 17,500 steps | Add 500 steps per day |

If you've been completely inactive, I want you to *phase in* activity. That means you will work at your own pace for as long as you need to. To phase in cardio, I recommend that, for the first 4 to 6 weeks, you shoot to do cardio at least three times a week (five or more times is optimal). See page 132 on ideas on how to do this. If you're already active, see page 136 for tips on how to crank up your workout.

**2. Perform resistance training two or three times a week for at least 30 minutes at a time, preferably 45 minutes.** Women usually understand why they need cardio: It burns fat. What they don't always get is why they need to lift weights. Well, it's pretty simple: You can't remove weight unless you lift weight. Let me give you my come-to-heaven lecture about the benefits of weight training.

Resistance training increases your muscular strength and endurance, boosts your energy, improves your balance and flexibility, and maintains or even builds bone density. It also powers up your metabolism, transforming your muscles into powerful fat burners. (Get this: Although a weight-training newbie burns 150 to 250 calories in one 45-minute session, her more muscular sister burns 300 to 400 calories in the same amount of time.) Lifting weights will also firm and shape your body, allowing you to fit into smaller sizes as it optimizes your body composition.

If you're new to weights, you'll need to learn how to do the exercises correctly (also known as "form"). The exercise descriptions in Appendix A also include handy tips to ensure that you follow proper form.

Most women haven't had much experience hoisting weights. That's why I recommend consulting a trainer to get instruction on proper form and how to lift safely so you won't get hurt. Getting expert guidance is especially important if you're over 35.

If you plan to join a gym, or are already a member, I suggest that you photocopy the exercises in Appendix A, take them to the gym, and ask a trainer to demonstrate the proper form for each exercise. (Always ask for advice if you are not sure about certain exercises.) Trainers at the gym are usually pretty good about providing you with quality advice, sometimes for free. You may have to schedule an appointment, but it's worth doing. I'd even recommend that you schedule a session with a trainer if you plan to work out at home.

If you'd still like to start with cardio and phase in the weights when you feel ready, that's fine. Didn't I tell you that this was a flexible program?

**3. Cross-train with yoga, Pilates, or other activities that help maintain or build flexibility and balance.** If you maintain your flexibility and balance now, you'll safeguard what doctors call functional independence—the ability to dress, get to the bathroom, and just generally take care of yourself as you grow

*(continued on page 134)*

## Go for the Burn

This chart shows you how many calories you can burn *per minute* while performing 35 popular forms of cardio activity. Notice that the heavier you are, the more you'll burn. So if you're around 150 pounds, you'll burn 330 calories in 30 minutes on an elliptical trainer. How cool is that?

| Activity | 100 lb | 125 lb | 150 lb | 175 lb | 200 lb | 225 lb | 250 lb | 275 lb | 300 lb |
|---|---|---|---|---|---|---|---|---|---|
| **Gym Activities** | | | | | | | | | |
| Aerobics, low-impact | 4 | 6 | 7 | 8 | 9 | 10 | 11 | 12 | 13 |
| Aerobics, step, low-impact | 6 | 7 | 8 | 10 | 11 | 13 | 14 | 15 | 17 |
| Aerobics, water | 3 | 4 | 5 | 6 | 6 | 7 | 8 | 9 | 10 |
| Bicycling, stationary (moderate) | 6 | 7 | 8 | 10 | 11 | 13 | 14 | 15 | 17 |
| Circuit training, general | 6 | 8 | 10 | 11 | 13 | 14 | 16 | 18 | 19 |
| Elliptical trainer | 7 | 9 | 11 | 13 | 14 | 16 | 18 | 20 | 22 |
| Rowing, stationary | 6 | 7 | 8 | 10 | 11 | 13 | 14 | 15 | 17 |
| Ski machine (general) | 8 | 10 | 11 | 13 | 15 | 17 | 19 | 21 | 23 |
| Stairstepper, general | 5 | 6 | 7 | 8 | 10 | 11 | 12 | 13 | 14 |
| Stretching (yoga) | 3 | 4 | 5 | 6 | 6 | 7 | 8 | 9 | 10 |
| Weight lifting, general | 2 | 3 | 4 | 4 | 5 | 5 | 6 | 7 | 7 |
| Weight lifting, vigorous | 5 | 6 | 7 | 8 | 10 | 11 | 12 | 13 | 14 |
| **Training/Sports Activities** | | | | | | | | | |
| Bicycling 12–13.9 mph | 6 | 8 | 10 | 11 | 13 | 14 | 16 | 18 | 19 |
| Bowling | 2 | 3 | 4 | 4 | 5 | 5 | 6 | 7 | 7 |
| Dancing: disco, ballroom, square | 5 | 6 | 7 | 8 | 9 | 10 | 11 | 12 | 13 |

| Activity | 100 lb | 125 lb | 150 lb | 175 lb | 200 lb | 225 lb | 250 lb | 275 lb | 300 lb |
|---|---|---|---|---|---|---|---|---|---|
| Frisbee | 2 | 3 | 4 | 4 | 5 | 5 | 6 | 7 | 7 |
| Golf (carrying clubs) | 5 | 6 | 7 | 8 | 9 | 10 | 11 | 12 | 13 |
| Ice skating, general | 6 | 7 | 8 | 10 | 11 | 13 | 14 | 15 | 17 |
| Hiking, cross-country | 5 | 6 | 7 | 8 | 10 | 11 | 12 | 13 | 14 |
| Horseback riding, general | 3 | 4 | 5 | 6 | 6 | 7 | 8 | 9 | 10 |
| Inline skating | 6 | 7 | 8 | 10 | 11 | 13 | 14 | 15 | 17 |
| Martial arts (judo, karate, etc.) | 8 | 10 | 12 | 14 | 16 | 18 | 20 | 22 | 24 |
| Race walking | 6 | 7 | 8 | 9 | 10 | 12 | 13 | 14 | 16 |
| Running 5 mph (12-min mile) | 6 | 8 | 10 | 11 | 13 | 14 | 16 | 18 | 19 |
| Skiing, downhill | 5 | 6 | 7 | 8 | 10 | 11 | 12 | 13 | 14 |
| Swimming, general | 5 | 6 | 7 | 8 | 10 | 11 | 12 | 13 | 14 |
| Tai chi | 3 | 4 | 5 | 6 | 6 | 7 | 8 | 9 | 10 |
| Tennis, general | 6 | 7 | 8 | 10 | 11 | 13 | 14 | 15 | 17 |
| Volleyball, general | 2 | 3 | 4 | 4 | 5 | 5 | 6 | 7 | 7 |
| Walking 4 mph (15 min/mile) | 4 | 5 | 5 | 6 | 7 | 8 | 9 | 10 | 11 |
| Walking 3.5 mph (17 min/mile) | 3 | 4 | 5 | 6 | 6 | 7 | 8 | 9 | 10 |
| **Gardening Activities** | | | | | | | | | |
| Digging, spading dirt | 4 | 5 | 6 | 7 | 8 | 9 | 10 | 11 | 12 |
| Gardening, general | 4 | 5 | 5 | 6 | 7 | 8 | 9 | 10 | 11 |
| Mowing lawn (push or power) | 4 | 5 | 5 | 6 | 7 | 8 | 9 | 10 | 11 |
| Sacking grass or leaves | 3 | 4 | 5 | 6 | 6 | 7 | 8 | 9 | 10 |

older. You'll also reduce your risk of hip-shattering falls. Yoga, Pilates, and tai chi fit the bill.

And talk about stress relief! My patients find that these slow, controlled forms of mind-body movements are very calming and improve their ability to cope with stress. Studies have shown that when women do yoga on a daily basis, the stress hormone cortisol decreases and stays down throughout the day. Controlling cortisol levels is vital to achieving optimally functioning hormone and immune systems.

Yoga, Pilates, and tai chi can be done with moderate or quite vigorous intensity. You don't need to take a class unless you want to (and many of my patients do). Instead, there are wonderful videos and DVDs available for home use. To start out, you can pick and choose from the yoga positions and Pilates moves in the "Stretches" section of Appendix A starting on page 194.

## GETTING THE MOST FROM YOUR BODY-*FOR*-LIFE FOR WOMEN TRAINING METHOD

Now that I've given you the basic Body-*for*-LIFE for Women Training Method template, I encourage—expect!—you to make it your own. Who knows your habits, temperament, and schedule better than you do?

To customize your training, consider the questions below. Then troubleshoot potential trouble spots and brainstorm solutions—even before you begin your training. Remember, ladies, success depends on your ability to plan and regroup!

• Will you join a gym or work out at home?

• Are you a morning person or a night owl?

• What kinds of physical activity intrigue you—or completely turn you off?

• Is your schedule comfortably predictable or out of control? Does it include frequent disruptions to care for kids or an aging parent, or frequent business travel?

• Do you prefer to exercise alone, with one other person, or in a group?

• Do you have previous injuries—a bad back, a bum knee or ankle—that preclude certain types of exercise?

Answering these questions will help you create a program that works for *you*. Here are some other suggestions that will help set you on the path to your own transformation.

## ADD SOME "VITAMIN I"

The latest fitness research shows that when it comes to burning fat and building muscle, it's not just about how long you spend walking on the treadmill or hefting dumbbells. Equally important is how hard you work—in other words, the *intensity* of your effort. I call it vitamin I.

It drives me absolutely crazy when I walk into a gym and see a woman on a treadmill walking 2½ miles an hour or lifting bitty little 2-pound dumbbells when it's obvious that she can walk faster or lift a lot more. It drives me even battier when I hear her in the locker room after her "workout," complaining that she just can't shed those extra pounds. If this sounds like you, listen up: Ladies, add some vitamin I! These tips can help you figure out your "dosage."

**Rate your effort.** When you exercise, your heart beats faster to meet your body's demand for more blood and oxygen. The harder you work out, the faster your heart will beat. Fitness experts use an objective measure of exercise intensity: maximum heart rate, or MHR, which requires using a heart monitor or taking your pulse. There is, however, a simpler way to gauge intensity: the rate of perceived exertion (RPE). The RPE is simply your subjective perception of how hard you're working.

To determine RPE, you use a scale of 0 to 10, with 10 being the highest intensity. Sitting quietly would be a 0; walking at a strolling pace rates a 3. And your rate isn't what you *think* you should feel; it's what you actually feel. Most people should exercise between an RPE of 5 (moderate) and 7 (strong).

**Remember that intensity is relative.** The intensity of your effort should depend on your general health and physical condition. For an unfit woman, moderate intensity might be 3 miles per hour on the treadmill at 0 incline. For a conditioned athlete, it might be running 5 miles per hour on an incline of 3 or 4.

No matter how high—or low—your RPE is, you have to sweat to get the benefits of exercise. There's no way around it: Intensity is the key to achieving those dramatic

### For Advanced Exercisers: Ramping It Up

If you're an intermediate or advanced exerciser and want to ramp up the *intensity* of your current cardio program, do any one or a combination of the following:

- Increase the speed of your cardio: walks, runs, bike rides, hikes, or swims.

- Increase the resistance or level of difficulty on your outdoor or stationary bike, elliptical trainer, or stepper, or swim with flippers.

- Raise the incline of your treadmill or elliptical trainer, or add hill work to your outdoor walking, running, biking, or hiking.

- Cross-train with two or more cardio programs.

To rev up your weight workout:

- Increase the weight level gradually and under appropriate supervision to challenge your muscle to become stronger, build more muscle fibers, and burn more fat.

- Mix up your workout, intermingling weights with bands, tubing, and machines.

- Don't get stuck in a rut doing the same exercises. For example, mix up the single dumbbell biceps curls with hammer curls.

- Try doing supersets, when you do one set followed immediately by another same-muscle exercise to fatigue.

- Train for a marathon, triathlon, or century (100-mile bike ride). Though demanding, this type of high-intensity training can bring you to an astounding level of physical and emotional transformation.

"after" photos. In fact, the women in the pictures may have been pushing their intensity beyond moderate, which may be part of the reason behind their rapid results. (And they've obviously sustained their efforts, too!)

As you become more fit, you'll be able to ramp up the intensity of your workout, burn even more calories, achieve higher levels of fitness, and get your workout done in a shorter period of time. More results, less time—what a deal!

**Start low and slow.** The Body-*for*-LIFE for Women Training Method asks that you work at an intensity that challenges you but that you can comfortably manage for the length of your workout. If you've received a clean bill of health from your doctor, I recommend that you work out at a moderate level of intensity, defined as walking a mile in 15 to 20 minutes, or a speed of roughly 3 to 4 miles per hour. On the RPE scale, you'd be slightly out of breath but still able to carry on a conversation. What's moderate intensity in resistance training? If you're sweating throughout your lifting, you're golden.

**Listen to your body.** Don't try high-intensity workouts without trainer-assisted guidance. Let your body guide your effort; neither push it too hard nor let it off too easily. It's all about continuously challenging yourself, reaching for the next level, doing more than dreaming about a powerful and fit body, but achieving your goal.

## PLAN FOR CARDIO SUCCESS

There are tons of books on how to walk, run, cycle, climb the Himalayas. I don't care what you do, as long as you do it for 30 minutes, 3 to 5 days a week. So choose an activity and go for it! (For cardio ideas, remember to check out the huge chart on page 132.) Readers of the original *Body*-for-*LIFE* will recall the 20-Minute Aerobics Solution. This high-intensity approach may be a bit challenging for beginners, but it is another alternative. (See www.bodyforlife.com for more details on this method.)

I will say one thing, though. To lose fat and increase your aerobic capacity, I recommend that you plan your workout around FIT principles. FIT stands for Frequency (times per week you work out), Intensity (the speed or amount of resistance you use), and Time (how long you perform the workout). As you become more fit, you can play with the FIT formula. For example, you might choose to increase intensity while maintaining time and frequency, or maintain intensity and time but increase frequency. (Just don't increase all three at the same time.)

I'm a stickler for warmups and cooldowns, which loosen up your muscles, lower the chance of injuries, and safely increase and reduce your heart rate before and after your workout. To maximize your cardio, keep these other recommendations in mind.

**Consider a pre-breakfast workout.** If you can, do your cardio before breakfast. Cardio on an empty stomach forces your body to tap into its stored body fat for energy.

**Start off slow and easy.** Gradually, over a period of weeks, you may increase any one of the following: the frequency of your workouts, the length of your workouts, or the level of their intensity. Never increase all three at once, and listen to your body—if it doesn't feel good, don't push it.

**Vary your cardio options.** For example, if you usually jog, try rowing or cycling. Switching your cardio activity doesn't just keep your workouts interesting; it challenges your body, too. Doing the same cardio routine over and over eventually can slow fat removal.

**Stretch before and after your workout.** This includes your calves, quadriceps (the large muscle in the front of your thighs), and hamstrings (the muscle in the back of your thighs). If you don't stretch, believe me, you'll feel it 5 minutes into your workout!

**Always warm up and cool down.** Three to 5 minutes of walking or marching in place before and after your workout helps bump your heart rate up, to prepare it for exertion, and ease it back to normal.

**Try cardio intervals.** As your fitness increases, try incorporating intervals into your cardio routine. Intervals are short bursts of intense exercise that are followed by periods of low-intensity activity. In its most basic form, interval training might involve walking for 1 minute, jogging for 30 seconds, and alternating this pattern throughout your workout. Base the length of your intervals on how you feel.

## REAP THE REWARDS OF STRENGTH TRAINING

Now, let's turn our attention to the secret weapon of the Body-*for*-LIFE for Women Training Method: weight training. Sure, cardio burns fat. But if you really want to transform your body, you have to add weight training.

Today, about 39 million Americans lift weights—a 62 percent increase since the 1970s—and a good portion of them are women. As you can see from the inside covers of this book, the transformations are breathtaking. Instead of allowing inactivity and gravity to take over, these women lost body fat, gained muscle, and toned and tightened their bodies from head to toe. That's because fat takes up much more space than muscle—about five times the space, in fact. So the more muscle you build, the smaller you'll look.

That's right—smaller. You may be fearful of "bulking up," but trust me: you won't. Though most women will experience a 20 to 40 percent increase in muscular strength after several months of resistance training, just like men, women just don't have enough of the hormones that would allow them to look like the Incredible Hulk.

Muscles don't get stronger in the gym—they get stronger after your workout is over. During your weight-training workouts, you will slightly damage your muscle fibers, causing microscopic tears in the muscle tissue. This damage to the muscles repairs itself only between workouts, and that's when muscle growth occurs. (In fact, when you train with weights, you actually use stored body fat to fuel the growth of your muscles!) You can help this repair process by fueling your body with the proper nutrients and getting adequate rest.

If you're a beginner, review the tips below right before you begin to lift, so that you'll have these critical principles and Body-*for*-LIFE for Women Training Method specifics in the front of your mind. With time, you'll follow them automatically. (Even if you've been lifting weights for a while, it can't hurt to review them.)

**Learn your reps and sets.** Whether you work out at home or join a gym, you'll need to know some basic terms. One *rep,* or repetition, describes one complete exercise. For example, one biceps curl is one rep. A *set* is a specific number of repetitions. On this program, you'll be doing three sets of each exercise. With each set, you'll increase the weight and reduce the repetitions. Do from 12 to 20 reps for your first set, from 12 to 15 reps for the second set, and from 8 to 10 reps for the third set.

**Get your motor running.** Take 5 to 10 minutes to walk briskly, do jumping jacks, or march or jog in place. If you do an aerobic workout in addition to resistance training, you can do the aerobics first, in place of a warmup.

**Pick the right weight.** If you can't lift the weight in good form 8 times, it's too heavy. If you can easily lift the weight more than 12 times, it's too light. Pick one in between.

**Alternate training between the upper and lower body.** For example, one week, you might train the upper body on Monday, the lower body on Wednesday, and the upper body on Friday. The next week, train the lower body on Monday, the upper body on Wednesday, and the lower body on Friday. Alternating between upper-body and lower-body workouts gives your muscles sufficient time to recover between workouts. And recovery is essential, because it's during rest that your muscles grow stronger.

**Shoot for two exercises per body part.** Perform two exercises for each major muscle group of the upper and lower body. The upper body includes chest, shoulders, back, triceps, and biceps. The lower body includes quadriceps, hamstrings, and calves. I suggest that you train your abs after your lower-body workout. Because you're training fewer muscle groups (compared with the upper-body routine), you'll have more time to fit them into your workout.

**Don't wait to exhale.** Many women who lift weights (experienced as well as in-experienced) hold their breath while they lift, which can cause their blood pressure to spike. Make it a point to exhale when you lift the weight or do the crunch and in-hale as you lower the weight or return to the starting position.

**Slow it down.** If it's worth doing, it's worth doing right. Fast, jerky movements can cause injury and force you to use momentum, rather than muscle, to lift the weight. Slow, controlled movements are safer and take more effort, so you get more benefit. Take 2 seconds to lift the weight, pause for 2 seconds, and then take another 2 seconds to lower the weight.

**Rest between sets.** Your muscles need time to recover between sets. So, for each muscle group, rest 1 minute between each set and 2 minutes before starting the next muscle group.

**Perfect your form.** Good form helps prevent injury and helps you get the most benefit from lifting. To watch your form, stand in front of a full-length mirror. (At a gym, mirrors are everywhere. If you're working out at home, get yourself an inexpensive full-length mirror at a discount department store.) Check that your wrists are straight—not bent backward or forward—and that you are doing the exercise precisely as it is shown.

**Pay attention to posture.** Whether you're sitting or standing when you lift, keep your back, neck, and head straight to prevent muscle strain and injury. If you're standing up, stand tall but relaxed. If you're seated, sit up straight with your feet flat on the floor.

**Be kind to your joints.** When you lock a joint, the joint bears the stress of the weight, not the muscle. To prevent joint pain, end the move just short of locking your knees or elbows.

**Take a day off.** Your muscles need at least a day to rest between training sessions. It's during that time that your muscles get stronger. That's because lifting weights causes tiny tears in the muscle tissue. As your muscles repair that damage, they become stronger.

**Work through soreness.** Ladies, if you haven't trained with weights before, there's no way around it—you're going to be stiff and sore for the first few weeks. We're talking *moderate* discomfort; you may wince as you walk down stairs or when you reach for the top shelf. This post-workout pain and inflammation, called delayed onset muscle soreness (DOMS), is caused by those tiny muscle tears I just mentioned. But the pain is worth it—it's this process of breakdown and repair that will build your Body-*for*-LIFE.

Don't increase the amount of weight until the soreness subsides. Generally speaking, DOMS peaks at about 2 days after a workout and dissipates on its own within a week.

**But don't ignore severe pain.** Muscle, joint, or ligament injuries are more painful than DOMS and last longer than a week. If the pain is sharp and severe, or doesn't fade within a week, seek medical treatment.

**Remember your vitamin I.** As you get more comfortable with the weights, ramp up the intensity of your workout to optimize your strength, tone, and muscular curves.

## THE BODY-*FOR*-LIFE FOR WOMEN PROGRAM SEGMENTS

You know the ground rules. Now let's put it all together. The Body-*for*-LIFE for Women Training Method is based on two segments. The first is a 12-week Weight Removal Segment, which can be repeated as many times as you wish until you reach your goal weight. (The second is the Weight Maintenance Segment, which we'll discuss in a bit.)

How should you determine your goal weight? First, check out "Your Ideal Weight" on page 142 and "Factors That May Affect Your Weight Loss" on page 143. They'll give you some sense of what a reasonable, attainable weight might be, given your height and personal circumstances. Then, ask yourself two questions.

## Your Ideal Weight

One logical question is, how much *should* you weigh? I suggest that you start with 100 pounds for the first 5 feet of you and add 5 pounds for every inch over that. So if you're 5 feet 6 inches, your ideal weight would be 130 pounds (plus or minus 13 pounds—10 percent—to account for different body frames).

A word about "ideal" weight: Your goal is to eliminate Toxic Fat, optimize your muscle mass, and remove as much body fat as possible. That may take you to within 20 to 30 pounds of your ideal body weight. So if you have 100 pounds to remove and you manage to remove 70, you may not be at your "ideal weight." But I'll tell you one thing: If you're fitter, and you've reduced your risk of disease by removing Toxic Weight, I'm thrilled! You've accomplished a truly remarkable feat and helped save your own life.

| Height | Ideal Weight (lb) |
|--------|-------------------|
| 5' | 100 |
| 5'1" | 105 |
| 5'2" | 110 |
| 5'3" | 115 |
| 5'4" | 120 |
| 5'5" | 125 |
| 5'6" | 130 |
| 5'7" | 135 |

| Height | Ideal Weight (lb) |
|--------|-------------------|
| 5'8" | 140 |
| 5'9" | 145 |
| 5'10" | 150 |
| 5'11" | 155 |
| 6' | 160 |
| 6'1" | 165 |
| 6'2" | 170 |

1. Thinking back over my adult life, at what weight—or what clothing size—did I look and feel healthiest and happiest?

2. Is getting to that weight again realistic? Yes, if you've held that weight before by following a healthy lifestyle. No, if it involves starving yourself to fit into your

---

**Factors That May Affect Your Weight Loss**

• **Your age:** Once you hit 40, removing body fat becomes a tad more challenging. However, it's completely doable, and you're gonna do it!

• **Your weight:** If you are currently 50 to 100 pounds overweight, don't expect to remove all of it in 12 weeks. Plan on a 6- to 24-pound weight removal for every 12-week segment.

• **Your hormonal status:** If you have a tough time with PMS, have recently had a child or are currently taking fertility medications, or are currently perimenopausal, hormonal fluctuations may affect your appetite and hunger. You'll need to pay more attention to staying consistent with your nutrition and training programs.

• **Your level of fitness:** If you are starting from square one, be patient; your body needs time to ramp up to speed. If you used to be active, your Body-*for*-LIFE may emerge more quickly than you think.

• **Your physical health:** If you have a medical condition that interferes with your ability to be as active as you'd like (you have a bum knee or arthritis, for example, or are recovering from surgery), you need to factor these into your weight-removal equation by picking a lower activity factor. Ditto if you are on medications that slow weight loss, such as hormone therapy, tamoxifen, certain antidepressants, beta-blockers, and prednisone.

---

high-school wardrobe and you are in Milestone 3 or 4. You have to have held that weight comfortably, without unreasonable effort.

Once you've arrived at a reasonable goal weight, you'll have a good idea of how many Weight Removal Segments you're looking at. Generally speaking, one Weight Removal Segment will suffice if you have up to 20 pounds to remove; to remove more, you'll probably need to do back-to-back segments. Depending on your current weight, you can reasonably expect to remove from 6 to 24 pounds in one Weight Removal Segment, which equates to about $1/2$ to 2 pounds per week. This range gives you plenty of wiggle room, allowing you to go all out on the program or take it more slowly. Either way, you're a success—any weight removed or muscle gained is wonderful.

When you hit your goal weight, you'll enter the second segment—Weight Maintenance. You can stay at Maintenance indefinitely, perhaps even for the rest of your life. But you also can slip into the Maintenance Segment *before* you reach goal weight, to maintain weight you've already removed without trying to lose more. I call this "treading weight," and it's a great way to keep the progress you've made in the face of illness, injury, or a rough patch at home or at work. (More about Maintenance and treading weight in a moment.)

Whether your goal is to remove 15 pounds or 50, be realistic. Don't expect it'll be easy to remove 2 pounds per week when you have only 10 to go. It's likely and perfectly normal that your weight removal will slow as you progress, because you have less to remove. Unfortunately, the dreaded plateau can happen to almost every woman: As you remove weight, your body's metabolism—the rate at which your body burns calories—often slows down. You're in luck, though, because increasing your physical activity by even 10 to 15 minutes a day—or changing your exercise routine—can help you bust through a plateau and kick-start your weight removal once again. Though hitting a plateau can be intensely frustrating, take heart: It means that you have less fat to remove, which is why it won't budge as easily. Besides, weight removed slowly and safely is more likely to stay gone.

Another thing to bear in mind: The women you see on the inside covers of this book removed from 20 to 30 pounds over a 12-week period with careful eating and consistent, high-intensity workouts. What's more, many of these pictures represent these women's *last* Weight Removal Segment—several of these ladies started their original Body-*for*-LIFE program with much more excess weight. If you have more than 30 pounds to remove, use their transformations to inspire yourself, but please don't compare yourself with them. Instead, draw encouragement from their "after-after" photos—evidence that this plan truly is sustainable!

Whether you're new to working out, an elite athlete, or anything in between, the Body-*for*-LIFE for Women Training Method will work for you because it is a program for every stage of your life. It will work no matter what the circumstances: after a pregnancy or surgery, after breaking a leg and gaining 10 pounds, whatever. So if there are periods in your life when you regain a few pounds, you'll know exactly what to do to remove them again. The key is to reenter the Body-*for*-LIFE for Women Training Method as soon as possible.

---

**How Are You Doing? Two (Other) Methods to Measure Your Progress**

Because muscle weighs more than fat, you may find that you drop a pants size or two while the number on your scale stays the same—or even inches up. Don't panic! Instead, chart your progress using these methods.

**Option 1: The Tape Measure Method.** Every 4 weeks, using a cloth tape measure, measure the following:

• Across your breasts

• Around the widest part of your upper arm

• Across your waist at belly button height

• Across the widest part of your abdomen (the menopot)

• Around the widest part of your buttocks

• Around the widest part of your thigh (about midthigh)

• Around the middle of your calf

**Option 2: The Clothes-O-Meter.** Pick out a tight piece of clothing that you can get on but can't yet fully button or zip. That's your clothes-o-meter, and it's a great way to monitor your progress. Hang it outside the closet, so you see it every day. Every week, *before* you hop on your scale, first pull on your clothes-o-meter and see how it fits. If it zips up better, you've dropped body fat—and clothing size!—and possibly have built a bit of muscle. So whatever the scale says, you know you're doing well.

---

**Body Fat: What's Healthy, What's Not**

For the average adult woman, the healthy range of body fat is shown below.

| Age | Healthy Range |
|-----|---------------|
| 18–39 | 21–32% |
| 40–59 | 23–33% |
| 60–79 | 24–35% |

---

## BEGINNING YOUR FIRST SEGMENT

Are you ready to begin? Start by selecting Day 1 of your first segment. I suggest *today*, because there's no better day to greet the rest of your life. On the other hand, if it's been a while since you worked out, you may require a bit of preparation to get ready, such as the following:

• Check your training shoes (be sure to invest in new ones every 6 months!).

• Pick exercise clothes you feel good wearing.

• Schedule your workouts so that last-minute craziness won't sidetrack you.

• Set up a meeting with a trainer.

• Purchase other equipment (if you're working out at home). (See "Getting Started: Your Equipment" for a full description of home gym needs.)

At the beginning and end of each 12-week Weight Removal Segment, you'll measure your progress by the change in your body composition—fat lost and muscle gained. I recommend that you purchase a body-fat analyzer (Tanita makes a good one, but there are others), which displays both your scale weight and body-fat percentage. These gadgets aren't completely accurate, but they're close enough. Or, if you belong to or plan to join a gym, you can have a trainer measure your body fat. (If they use skinfold calipers rather than a body-fat analyzer, be sure to remeasure every 12 weeks using the same trainer, under the same conditions.)

## Getting Started: Your Equipment

The equipment below is all you need to start this training program. You can either find these items in a gym or set up your own workout space at home. Any department store or large sporting goods store carries this stuff, and sometimes it's easier (and cheaper!) to do your workouts at home.

- Dumbbells. Not the kind with plates—too clunky. Opt for either the plastic-coated ones (two 10-pound dumbbells cost about $20) or the sleek, chrome kind (two 10-pounders for about $40). I recommend using 10-pound weights—again, it's all about *intensity*.

- A weight bench. Choose one that can be used flat and that also inclines. They start at around $50 and go up from there.

- An exercise mat ($20) for stretching exercises. It should be made of vinyl or a rubbery surface—you're going to sweat on it, remember—and long enough so that when you lie on it, there's mat above your head and below your feet.

- A stability ball ($12 to $25) for abdominal exercises. Using one deepens the effects of exercises such as situps, as you're forced to use more muscles. There are different balls for different heights, so be sure to pick the one that's right for you.

- Resistance tubing. These stretchy little numbers are terrific for getting in a workout when you're traveling and can't get to a gym. I recommend the Xertube, by Spri. Each color gives a different amount of resistance—light, medium, or heavy. Each band costs around $10.

- A full-length mirror to check and perfect your form.

- A pair of well-fitting training shoes. Replace them every 6 months.

- A sturdy chair with a waist-high back for stretching. You can also do triceps dips off the edge of the seat.

- High-energy music. Whatever you prefer—rock, disco, hip-hop—play it loud! Your energy level—and the intensity of your workout—will go way up. Burn or record a special workout CD or tape of favorite songs, or simply buy a workout CD.

You'll also measure your progress with two other low-tech methods: a tape measure and my clothes-o-meter (see page 145). So many women get hung up on the number on the scale, and if they're not seeing big changes there (because they haven't opened their eyes to other methods of measuring progress), they'll feel as if they've failed. But as I've said before, depending on scale weight alone is not an accurate way to gauge your progress, especially as you gain muscle with weight training. Even if your scale weight isn't dropping rapidly, you may be trimming inches, dropping dress sizes, and removing body fat. Lost inches and looser clothing will help convince you that the Body-*for*-LIFE for Women Training Method is working for you. Scale weight is just a small piece of the action. Your goal is to optimize your body composition.

Ladies, open your mind to other definitions of success. The beauty of the Body-*for*-LIFE program is that it's not just about "losing weight," it's about *gaining a life*—a new, better life, filled with perks: more energy, a more positive outlook, more weight lifted in the gym, more minutes or miles on the treadmill, more passion for life, more self-confidence and self-esteem. When you measure success beyond the scale, the benefits of the program seem limitless.

Once you've assembled your gear, gotten the all clear from your doctor, and selected a start date, go ahead and launch into the 12-week Weight Removal Segment, following the nutrition guidelines in part 4 and the physical activity guidelines in this part. Remember the Power Mind principles to keep you focused. Repeat the Weight Removal Segment until you've removed the amount of weight you want. When you hit your goal weight or want to tread weight, enter the Weight Maintenance Segment.

On the opposite page, you'll find a simple way to record your progress on the Body-*for*-LIFE for Women Training Method: The Weight Removal Segment Checklist. Use the checklist to get a snapshot of your progress every 4 weeks, and then when you reach the 12-week mark, at the beginning and end of every Weight Removal Segment. (If you're handy with a calculator, you might also wish to use the Alternate Weight Removal Segment Formula, in Appendix D, on page 226. It can help you determine the number of calories you should eat and burn in each Weight Removal Segment to ensure that you continue to remove weight.)

## The Weight Removal Segment Checklist

Fill out the following checklist every 4 weeks and/or at the beginning or end of every 12-week Weight Removal Segment.

Segment Number: _____          Week Number: _____

### BODY-FAT PERCENTAGE

Beginning of Segment: _____          End of Segment: _____

### CLOTHES-O-METER

Beginning of Segment: _____          End of Segment: _____

Looser _____ No change _____          Looser _____ No change _____

### MEASUREMENTS

**Chest**    Beginning of Segment: _____          End of Segment: _____

**Waist** (across belly button)

    Beginning of Segment: _____          End of Segment: _____

**Hip**    Beginning of Segment: _____          End of Segment: _____

**Thigh** (left, right)

    Beginning of Segment: _____ , _____          End of Segment: _____ , _____

### MENOPOT

Beginning of Segment: Smaller _____ No change _____

End of Segment: Smaller _____ No change _____

### SCALE WEIGHT

Beginning of Segment: _____          End of Segment: _____

### MOOD

Beginning of Segment: _____          End of Segment: _____

### ENERGY LEVELS

Beginning of Segment: _____          End of Segment: _____

### OVERALL QUALITY OF LIFE

Beginning of Segment: _____          End of Segment: _____

## MOVING INTO WEIGHT MAINTENANCE
## AND "TREADING WEIGHT"

You transition into the Weight Maintenance Segment for one of two reasons. The first reason: You're at goal weight—hooray!—and want to stay there. The second: You want to tread weight.

The Weight Maintenance Segment allows you to tread weight just as you tread water. Think of treading weight as a kind of break-glass-in-case-of-emergency tactic, when you're too stressed or overwhelmed to go on with the Body-*for*-LIFE for Women Training Method. It's a gift you give yourself—a gentle, loving "pause" that allows you to step back from more-aggressive weight removal and simply maintain what you've achieved until you feel you're ready to step back into the segments again. You can tread weight at any time during a Weight Removal Segment, even if you haven't yet achieved your goal weight.

To find out if you want to enter the Weight Maintenance Segment to tread weight, ask yourself these questions at any time during a Weight Removal Segment:

• Have I removed enough weight for now? Do I want to take a break from aggressive weight removal and maintain for a while before I reenter the Body-*for*-LIFE for Women Training Method?

• Is there too much stress in my life right now? Do I want to maintain "until the hurricane blows over," then return to the Weight Removal Segment?

If you answer yes to both questions, slip into a Weight Maintenance Segment and tread weight until you feel ready to return to the Weight Removal Segment. Don't beat yourself up about it either. After working the program and taking a few spins through the segments, you'll get really good at the regrouping thing, believe me!

On the Weight Maintenance Segment, you'll eat and burn the amount of calories to *stay at your current* weight, rather than to continue to remove weight. That means you can eat a little more than you would in a Weight Removal Segment, and/or exercise a little less. (The Alternate Weight Maintenance Segment Formula, in Appendix D, on page 228 can help you figure out how many calories to eat and burn to hold steady, neither gaining weight nor removing it. Remember, you don't have to count calories unless you want to.)

Now, let's be clear: Whether you're maintaining or treading weight, it's essential to get *some* physical activity and follow *some* nutrition plan. Take your cues from some real "successful losers"—the participants in the National Weight Control Registry, who have shed an average of 50 pounds and kept it off for many years. Here's how they said they maintain their weight loss.

- They eat five times a day, on average.

- They move their bodies on a regular basis—less than 9 percent said they could maintain their weight with diet alone.

- They don't skip meals, especially breakfast.

Other ways to follow the Weight Maintenance Segment might include the following:

**Keep a eye on "weight drift."** Once a week, use your clothes-o-meter and take your measurements; once a month, check your body-fat percentage. On the Weight Removal Segment, you're using the clothes-o-meter and your measurements to chart your progress. In the Weight Maintenance Segment, you're using them to keep on the alert for weight drift. Same tactic, different reason.

**Continue to use your Mind-Mouth-Muscle Daily Journal.** The folks in the National Weight Control Registry also maintain a food and/or activity log to keep them aware of their eating. Studies have shown that people who keep a food diary and monitor what they eat consume less than those who do not. In one study, researchers at the Center for Behavioral Medicine in Chicago followed 38 dieters (who'd already lost an average of 21 pounds) from 2 weeks before Thanksgiving until 2 weeks after New Year's to find out if keeping a food diary would help them maintain their weight loss through the holidays. The dieters who wrote down what they ate lost an average of 7 pounds more; those who didn't gained back an average of 3 pounds.

**Change up your cardio.** Even when you're in the Weight Maintenance Segment, you'll want your cardio workout to adhere to FIT principles, which comprise the essentials of training for health and fitness. So, during Maintenance, you might reduce your cardio sessions to two or three a week for 20 minutes but add or maintain intensity (which is what burns the most calories and is most beneficial for cardiovascular health). Some options: bike or hike instead of walking, or take an extra yoga class instead of heading for the treadmill or elliptical trainer.

**Lift at least once a week, preferably twice.** Some research shows that "detraining"—which is just a fancy word for losing fitness—can start in as little as *4 days* after your last workout. The good news? Research shows that muscle strength and size can be maintained with one or two weight-training sessions a week.

If you follow the Body-*for*-LIFE for Women Training Method faithfully, you *will* see results. And whether your motivation is to maintain or improve your health or to once again button your jeans, changing your body composition can change your life. Just ask Linda.

## THE PAYOFF: LINDA'S STORY

At the beginning of this part, I told you that exercise can change a woman's life. I hope I've convinced you that it's true. I also want you to believe that with enough courage and commitment and, yes, sweat, it can change *your* life. Read a story of transformation from one of my patients, Linda, a travel agent who lives in Virginia and also ran in the 2001 New York City Marathon with me.

*August 6, 2000. My 50th birthday. I'd been married for 21 years, had two children, and was 40 pounds overweight. Oh, and my husband had just informed me that he'd be leaving me when our youngest son graduated from high school—in 8 years.*

*Our marriage was unhappy. We had nothing in common except the kids. He liked to golf; I didn't. He liked hard rock music; I liked classical. He liked to drink; I didn't. Things were so awful between us that he didn't spend my 50th birthday with the kids and me. He played in a golf tournament instead.*

*That day, at 50, I decided that I didn't like my life and I was the only one who could change it. I also realized that when my husband left, I'd need to support myself.*

*The first thing to do, I decided, was to lose some weight to boost my self-confidence, so I would stand a better chance of landing a job. Back then, I was very underconfident. I didn't think I was good at anything, and I certainly didn't like the way I looked.*

*To launch my new life, I walked across the Golden Gate Bridge in San Francisco with my entire family, husband excepted. When I got home, I began to walk—around the block. Every day.*

*Three months later, during a phone conversation, my friend Cindy told me she had started seeing Dr. Peeke. Then she asked me if I would like to run a marathon.*

*I replied, "Actually, yes. I would."*

*I got a copy of* Fight Fat after Forty *and started following Dr. Peeke's advice as best I could. Cindy and I began training together. When we started, we could barely walk a mile on the treadmill. But my walking/running "dates" with Cindy kept me going. Actually, they kept both of us going.*

*The weight started coming off—a pound a week. My clothes were looser. I noticed that I wasn't as depressed. My self-esteem rose. Even my husband noticed my commitment to running.*

*I thought, "If I can keep this up and finish the New York City Marathon next November, I will have really accomplished something."*

*By March 2001, I had lost about 20 pounds. I kept running.*

*In July, I discovered that for the past 5 years, my husband had been having an affair with a family friend. I ran harder and faster. Running helped me get through our subsequent divorce proceedings amicably, for the sake of our sons.*

*That November, 40 pounds lighter, I ran/walked the New York City Marathon with the women in Dr. Peeke's group. During that race, I discovered that there was more to me than I knew.*

*At the 20-mile mark, I broke with the group, who were fatigued and had suffered injuries. I wanted to complete the race in under 6 hours, so I sped up.*

*I finished in 5 hours and 43 minutes. I was ecstatic. Even more so the next day, when the statistics in the* New York Times *showed that, in the last 6 miles of the race, I had passed over 1,000 runners. I'd run under 11-minute miles—for the first time since I'd begun my training.*

*Running has brought out a strength and courage and determination that I never knew I had. It taught me that I can endure disappointments and hardships. That I will not be crushed by life's curves. That I will survive. That I can accomplish any goal I set for myself.*

*This knowledge has changed my life.*

How about you? Are you ready to change *your* life?

## THE END OF THIS BOOK . . . AND THE BEGINNING OF YOUR JOURNEY

So there's the package. Mind, Mouth, and Muscle.

I have never, ever met a woman who didn't possess the Power Mind to transform

---

**Overview of the Body-*for*-LIFE for Women Training Method**

• Perform cardio—any planned activity that raises your heart rate for a sustained period of time, including walking, biking, cardio kickboxing, treadmill—*at least* three to five times a week for 30 minutes at a time.

• Lift weights two or three times a week for at least 30 minutes at a time. Alternate training the major muscles of the upper and lower body. For example, if you choose to lift three times one week, train the upper body on Monday, the lower body on Wednesday, and the upper body on Friday. The next week, train the lower body on Monday, the upper body on Wednesday, and the lower body on Friday. And so on.

• On weight-training days, perform two exercises for each major muscle group. On days you train your upper body, include chest, shoulders, back, triceps, and biceps. If it's a lower-body day, train your quadriceps, hamstrings, and calves. Train your abs after your lower body.

• Do three sets of each exercise. With each set, increase the weight and decrease your repetitions. Do 12 to 20 reps your first set, 12 to 15 reps the second set, and 8 to 10 reps the third and final set. For each muscle group, rest 1 minute between each set and 2 minutes before starting the next muscle group.

herself, mind and body. In fact, I have witnessed breathtaking mental and physical transformations in women who believed that they could do it—and did. When a woman's mind, body, and spirit unite, miracles happen. Her transformation becomes a gift that keeps on giving. She inspires other women, helps them to believe that they can have what she has and achieve what she's achieved.

If you've just finished the book, lay the groundwork for a successful start to your Challenge. De-junk your kitchen; stock your fridge and pantry with healthy, woman-friendly food. Put away the clothes hanging on your treadmill, dust off the dumbbells in your basement, and scope out a gym, a walking buddy, or perhaps a trainer to get you started. Make sure your shoes are in good shape, and if they're not, please invest in a new pair—you're going to need them! Photocopy the pages you need of the Mind-Mouth-Muscle Journals for your first 12-week Challenge.

*(continued on page 158)*

- Perform both cardio and weight training at the highest level of intensity that is comfortable for you. Your goal is to ramp up the intensity as your fitness level increases. Get an assessment by a fitness expert to make certain you're exercising at a safe and appropriate level for you.

- Cross-train to keep your metabolism humming.

- Progress through the Weight Removal Segments until you've removed the amount of weight you want (or until you want to tread weight). Then transition to the Weight Maintenance Segment. Should you gain weight, simply reenter the Weight Removal Segments until you've removed those extra pounds.

- Stretch before both cardio and weight training. Stretching helps you move freely during aerobic exercise, enables your muscles to build more strength when you lift weights, and helps you relax after a workout. (For stretching exercises, see page 194.)

- Warm up before both cardio and weight training. Warming up loosens your muscles and lowers the chance of injuries. To warm up, perform the same activity you plan to do but at a lower speed or intensity for 10 minutes, then go into your regular workout. At the end of your workout, reduce the intensity for 5 minutes. This cooldown will allow your muscles to relax and get your heart rate down slowly.

## The Body-*for*-LIFE for Women Training Method Schedule

Here's a sample training schedule for the next 12 weeks—and for the weeks and months after that. You can use it forever, throughout all of your Weight Removal and Weight Maintenance Segments. To get the most from it, however, make sure to increase the intensity of your efforts as your fitness level increases (as well as add extra cardio workouts). And don't forget to mix up your workouts! Go ahead—alternate your treadmill workout with cycling, or stairclimbing with jogging. Cross-training will challenge your body, help you avoid getting hurt from overusing certain muscles or repetitive motion, and keep boredom at bay. (*Note:* You can have your Free Day any day of the week—your choice. Just make sure you keep that time for yourself and really relax!)

|  | Monday | Tuesday |
|---|---|---|
| Week 1 | Day 1 Cardio (at least 30 minutes) | Day 2 Weights: Upper body |
| Week 2 | Day 8 Weights: Lower body/Abs | Day 9 Cardio (at least 30 minutes) |
| Week 3 | Day 15 Cardio (at least 30 minutes) | Day 16 Weights: Upper body |
| Week 4 | Day 22 Weights: Lower body/Abs | Day 23 Cardio (at least 30 minutes) |
| Week 5 | Day 29 Weights: Upper body | Day 30 Cardio (at least 30 minutes) |
| Week 6 | Day 36 Weights: Lower body/Abs | Day 37 Cardio (at least 30 minutes) |
| Week 7 | Day 43 Weights: Upper body | Day 44 Cardio (at least 30 minutes) |
| Week 8 | Day 50 Weights: Lower body/Abs | Day 51 Cardio (at least 30 minutes) |
| Week 9 | Day 57 Weights: Upper body | Day 58 Cardio (at least 30 minutes) |
| Week 10 | Day 64 Weights: Lower body/Abs | Day 65 Cardio (at least 30 minutes) |
| Week 11 | Day 71 Weights: Upper body | Day 72 Cardio (at least 30 minutes) |
| Week 12 | Day 78 Weights: Lower body/Abs | Day 79 Cardio (at least 30 minutes) |

| Wednesday | Thursday | Friday | Saturday | Sunday |
|---|---|---|---|---|
| Day 3 Cardio (at least 30 minutes) | Day 4 Weights: Lower body/Abs | Day 5 Cardio (at least 30 minutes) | Day 6 Weights: Upper body | Day 7 Free Day |
| Day 10 Weights: Upper body | Day 11 Cardio (at least 30 minutes) | Day 12 Weights: Lower body/Abs | Day 13 Cardio (at least 30 minutes) | Day 14 Free Day |
| Day 17 Cardio (at least 30 minutes) | Day 18 Weights: Lower body/Abs | Day 19 Cardio (at least 30 minutes) | Day 20 Weights: Upper body | Day 21 Free Day |
| Day 24 Weights: Upper body | Day 25 Cardio (at least 30 minutes) | Day 26 Weights: Lower body/Abs | Day 27 Cardio (at least 30 minutes) | Day 28 Free Day |
| Day 31 Weights: Lower body/Abs | Day 32 Cardio (at least 30 minutes) | Day 33 Weights: Upper body | Day 34 Cardio (at least 30 minutes) | Day 35 Free Day |
| Day 38 Weights: Upper body | Day 39 Cardio (at least 30 minutes) | Day 40 Weights: Lower body/Abs | Day 41 Cardio (at least 30 minutes) | Day 42 Free Day |
| Day 45 Weights: Lower body/Abs | Day 46 Cardio (at least 30 minutes) | Day 47 Weights: Upper body | Day 48 Cardio (at least 30 minutes) | Day 49 Free Day |
| Day 52 Weights: Upper body | Day 53 Cardio (at least 30 minutes) | Day 54 Weights: Lower body/Abs | Day 55 Cardio (at least 30 minutes) | Day 56 Free Day |
| Day 59 Weights: Lower body/Abs | Day 60 Cardio (at least 30 minutes) | Day 61 Weights: Upper body | Day 62 Cardio (at least 30 minutes) | Day 63 Free Day |
| Day 66 Weights: Upper body | Day 67 Cardio (at least 30 minutes) | Day 68 Weights: Lower body/Abs | Day 69 Cardio (at least 30 minutes) | Day 70 Free Day |
| Day 73 Weights: Lower body/Abs | Day 74 Cardio (at least 30 minutes) | Day 75 Weights: Upper body | Day 76 Cardio (at least 30 minutes) | Day 77 Free Day |
| Day 80 Weights: Upper body | Day 81 Cardio (at least 30 minutes) | Day 82 Weights: Lower body/Abs | Day 83 Cardio (at least 30 minutes) | Day 84 Free Day |

Check in with your doctor to get a clean bill of health, and then find inspiration in the real-life success stories that begin on page 229. Pick a date, and go for it!

Your dream of living well, of feeling and looking great, can be a reality if you can allow your Power Mind to guide you. I want to be a part of your transformation, and I want to hear from you as you accept and live the Challenge (www.drpeeke.com).

As one of my patients said after completing her first 12-week Weight Removal Segment, "This was the first 12 weeks of the rest of my life." Now it's your turn.

# *Exercise Guide*

*Appendix A*

## MAJOR MUSCLE GROUPS

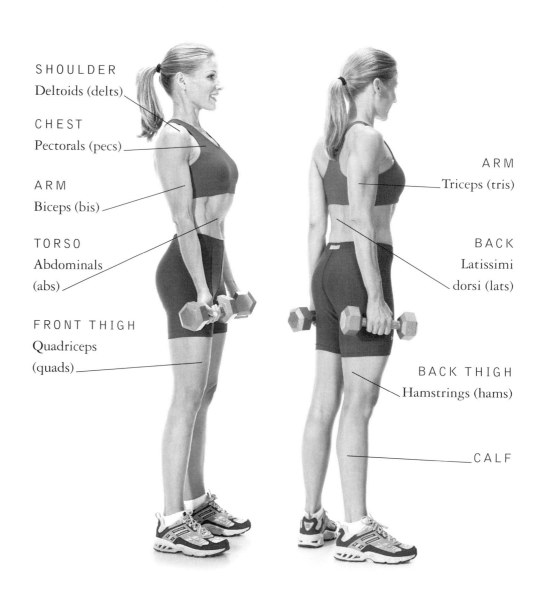

SHOULDER
Deltoids (delts)

CHEST
Pectorals (pecs)

ARM
Biceps (bis)

TORSO
Abdominals
(abs)

FRONT THIGH
Quadriceps
(quads)

ARM
Triceps (tris)

BACK
Latissimi
dorsi (lats)

BACK THIGH
Hamstrings (hams)

CALF

## DUMBBELL CHEST PRESS

**Starting Position:** Lie on your back on a bench, holding a dumbbell in each hand. Bring the weights to a point just above your shoulders, palms facing toward your feet and elbows out.

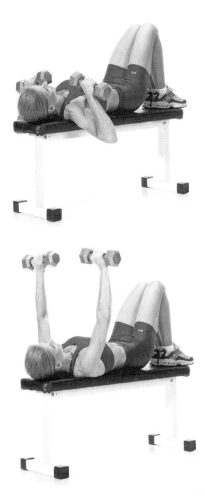

**The Exercise:** Press the weights straight up until they're right over your collarbone (not over your face or belly). Then slowly lower them to the starting position, feeling the stretch in your chest muscles as your elbows drop below the level of the bench.

**TIP**

*Don't let the dumbbells sway back toward your head and over your face. Don't let your head rise off the bench throughout the exercise.*

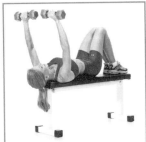

## INCLINE DUMBBELL PRESS

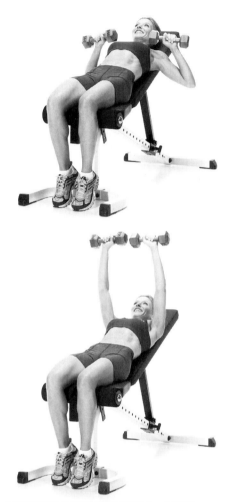

**Starting Position:** Sit on the edge of an incline bench, with the bench inclined at approximately a 30-degree angle. Pick up a dumbbell in each hand, place them on your thighs, and then, one at a time, position them at the base of your shoulders. Lean back and get firmly situated on the bench.

**The Exercise:** Press the weights up to a point over your upper chest, lifting them over your nose, and hold them there for a count of one. Then inhale deeply as you lower the weights to the starting position. Hold the weights in the bottom position for a brief count of one, and then exhale and drive them back up.

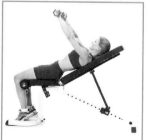

TIP

*If you feel the exercise more in your shoulders than in your upper chest, the bench angle is too steep.*

CHEST

## DUMBBELL FLY

**Starting Position:** Sit on the edge of a bench, with a dumbbell in each hand. Then lie back, keeping the dumbbells close to your chest. Bend your knees, and position your feet flat on the bench. Your hips and shoulders should be firmly situated on the bench. Press the weights straight up over your chest with your palms facing each other. Your elbows should be bent at a slight angle, as if you were hugging a ball.

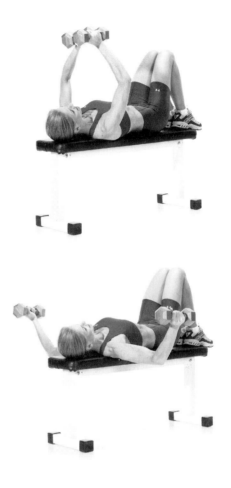

**The Exercise:** With your elbows slightly bent, begin to slowly lower the dumbbells. Then, keeping your elbows slightly bent, slowly lower the dumbbells out to the sides while inhaling deeply, until they are on a horizontal plane even with the bench. Really stretch those pecs, but don't lower the weights all the way to the floor.

Hold for a count of one, and then exhale while you lift the weights. Keep your arms just slightly bent at the elbows. And move the weights in an arc.

TIP

*Keep your elbows at the same angle throughout the exercise. Do not bend them more or straighten them as you work through the exercise; doing that would decrease the effectiveness of the exercise and possibly strain your shoulder muscles.*

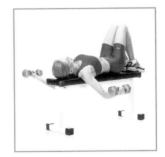

CHEST

## KNEE PUSHUP

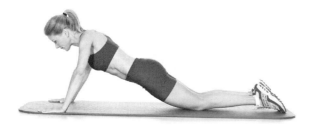

**Starting Position:** Kneel on all fours, your arms straight and shoulder-width apart and in line with your shoulders, your fingers facing forward. Your knees should be under your hips. Walk your hands forward about 6 inches; then press your hips forward until your body forms a straight line from your head to your hips.

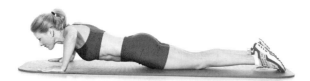

**The Exercise:** Contract your abdominal muscles and squeeze your shoulder blades together and down. Maintaining your starting position, bend your elbows out to the sides and lower your torso until your elbows are bent at a 90-degree angle and aligned with your shoulders. Contracting your chest and triceps to straighten your arms, return to the starting position without locking your elbows.

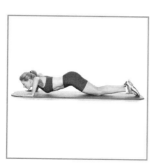

### TIP

*Keep your body in a straight line—do not sway your back.*

## FULL PUSHUP

**Starting Position:** Kneel on all fours, your arms slightly more than shoulder-width apart, your wrists in line with your shoulders, your fingers facing forward. Your knees should be in line with your hips. Contract your abdominal muscles and squeeze your shoulder blades together and down. Extend one leg at a time behind you so that you're supported on the balls of your feet and your body forms a straight line from your head to your heels. Look straight down.

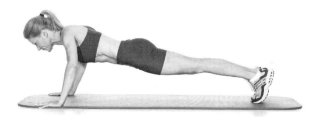

**The Exercise:** Maintaining your starting position, bend your elbows out to the sides and lower your torso toward the floor until your elbows are bent at a 90-degree angle and aligned with your shoulders. Contracting your chest and triceps to straighten your arms, return to the starting position without locking your elbows.

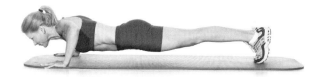

TIP

*Don't let your abs and hips sag as you lower yourself to the floor.*
*To prevent this, contract your glutes and leg muscles.*

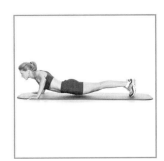

## SEATED DUMBBELL PRESS

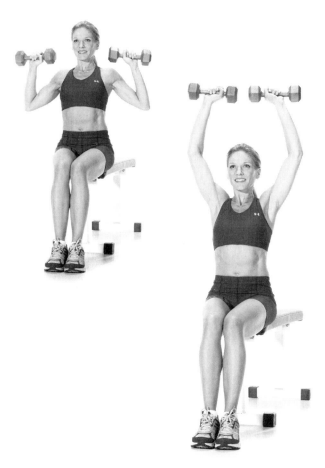

**Starting Position:** Sit on the end of a bench, with your feet flat on the floor. Hold a dumbbell in each hand at shoulder height, elbows out and palms facing forward.

**The Exercise:** Press the dumbbells up and in so they nearly touch above your head. Don't let the weights sway back and forth. Press the weights up until your arms are almost straight (with your elbows just short of locked). Then slowly lower the dumbbells to the starting position.

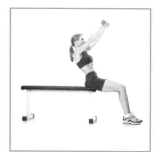

TIP

*Maintain good posture throughout this exercise. Do not lean backward. Look straight ahead with your chin up, shoulders squared, and chest high. Keep your arms in line with your ears so that you lift the weights straight over your head.*

SHOULDER

## FRONT RAISE

**Starting Position:** Stand with your feet shoulder-width apart, knees slightly bent, back straight, and abdominals contracted. Hold a dumbbell in each hand with your arms hanging down at the front of your thighs, palms facing in.

**The Exercise:** Keeping your wrists straight and your elbows slightly bent, raise your arms in front of you to shoulder height with your palms facing the floor. Hold; then slowly lower. To avoid swinging your arms or arching your back and using momentum to lift, try this move with your back against a wall. Or alternate one arm at a time.

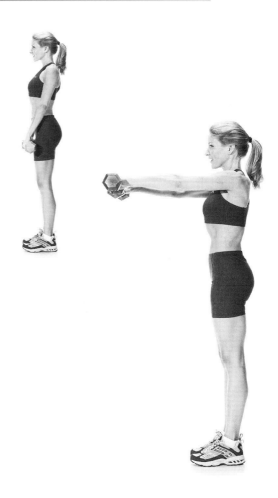

**TIP**

*Don't lean backward as you lift the weights. To get the proper form, balance your weight evenly between your toes and heels. Do not lift the weights beyond shoulder height.*

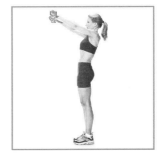

SHOULDER

## PRONE FLY

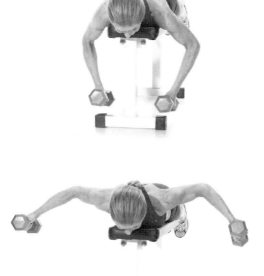

**Starting Position:** Lie facedown on a flat bench, with your chin just over the edge. Keep your legs together and straight. Pick up your dumbbells, one in each hand. Let your arms hang straight down, but keep your elbows slightly bent so that the dumbbells are slightly raised.

**The Exercise:** Squeeze your shoulder blades together and slightly elevate your chest. Now lift your arms up and out to your sides to shoulder level—no more. Your palms should be facing down. Pause; then slowly lower arms to the starting position.

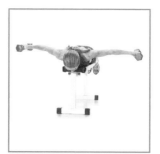

### TIP

*Don't lift your arms any higher than shoulder height or straighten your elbows—if you do, you may strain your shoulder or chest muscles.*

# SEATED DUMBBELL LATERAL RAISE

**Starting Position:** Sit on the end of a flat bench, your knees bent, your feet flat on the floor. Hold a dumbbell in each hand, and allow your arms to hang at your sides. Your palms should face inward, with thumbs facing forward.

**The Exercise:** Maintaining your posture, lift your arms up and out until they're parallel to the floor. Your palms should be facing down. Pause; then slowly lower your arms to the starting position.

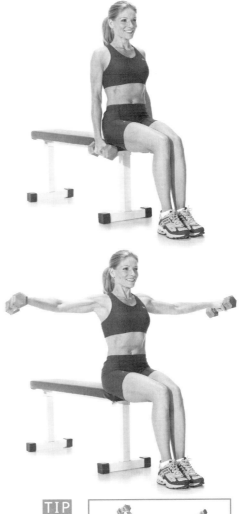

**TIP**

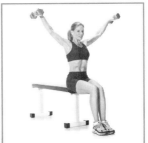

*Don't use momentum to get your arms above shoulder height—you could hurt your shoulder or rotator cuff muscles. If you find that you have to use momentum to lift the dumbbells, they're too heavy.*

SHOULDER

## STANDING DUMBBELL LATERAL RAISE

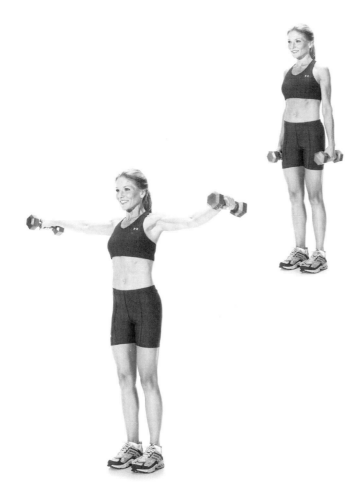

**Starting Position:** Stand with your feet about hip-width apart, your knees slightly bent, and your weight balanced between your toes and heels. Hold a dumbbell in each hand and allow your arms to hang by your sides. Your palms should face inward, with thumbs facing forward.

**The Exercise:** Maintaining your posture, lift your arms up and out to your sides until they're at shoulder height. Your palms should be facing down. Pause; then slowly lower your arms to the starting position.

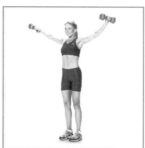

**TIP**

*Don't scrunch your shoulders above your ears. Keep your shoulders down and your chest lifted, and look straight ahead, with your chin level.*

SHOULDER

## ONE-ARM DUMBBELL ROW

**Starting Position:** Start with your right foot flat on the floor and your left knee resting on a flat bench; hold a dumbbell in your right hand. Then lean forward so you're supporting the weight of your upper body with your left arm on the bench. Your back should be almost parallel with the floor. Let your right arm hang straight down from your shoulder, with your palm turned in toward your body, your thumb facing forward.

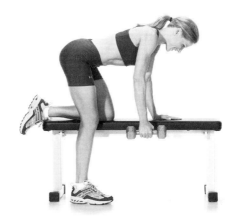

**The Exercise:** Pull your elbow back as far as it can go. The dumbbell should end up roughly parallel with your torso. After you've "rowed" the dumbbell up as far as you can, slowly lower it to the starting position.

After you complete the planned number of reps for your right arm, follow the same instructions for your left.

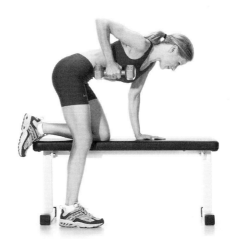

TIP

*Don't hunch or round your back. Keep it flat.*

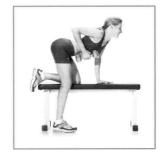

BACK

## DUMBBELL PULLOVER

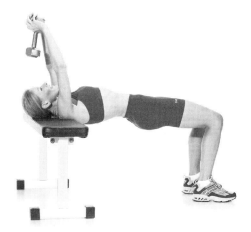

**Starting Position:** Pick up a dumbbell and hold it close to your chest as you position yourself on a flat bench. As you lie across the bench, be sure that only your upper back makes contact. Lift the weight overhead, and hold it (from its collar) at arm's length over your face.

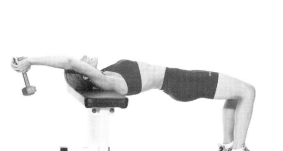

**The Exercise:** Without raising your hips, lower the dumbbell behind you in an arc while you breathe in very deeply. When you reach a fully stretched position, hold it for a quick count of one, and then raise the weight back up in an arc, exhaling deeply.

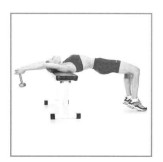

TIP

*Don't let your hips rise as you lower the dumbbell behind your head—keep your hips in the same low spot.*

BACK

## ONE-ARM CABLE ROW

**Starting Position:** Standing with your knees slightly bent, place resistance tubing under your feet. Cross the tubing and grasp the handles with your hands. Bend slightly forward at the waist, keeping a straight back. To help maintain proper form, press your chest forward and pull your shoulders back.

**The Exercise:** Pull one elbow up toward the ceiling. Make sure you retract your shoulder blade to perform the exercise properly. Your arm should remain close to your body throughout the exercise.

After you complete the planned number of reps for one arm, follow the same instructions for the other.

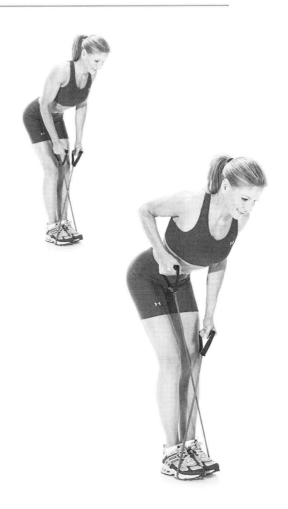

**TIP**

*With this exercise, form is important. Keep the tubing at midabdomen height, not chest height, and as you draw back your elbow, allow it to just brush your side.*

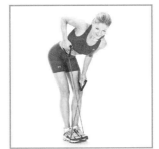

## BENCH DIP

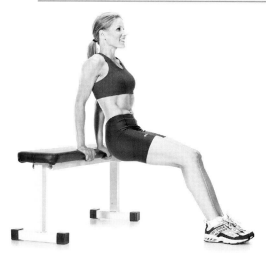

**Starting Position:** Stand with your back to a sturdy bench or chair. Bend your legs and place your hands on the front edge of the bench. Position your feet in front of you so most of your body weight is resting on your arms.

**The Exercise:** Keeping your elbows tucked against your sides, bend your arms and slowly lower your body until your upper arms are almost parallel to the floor. Your hips should drop straight down. Then straighten your arms and return to the starting position.

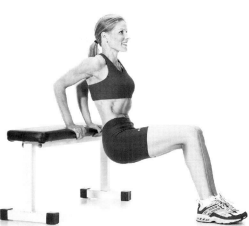

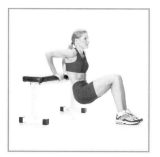

TIP

*Don't lower your body too far. That can stress your shoulders. Also, don't let your upper body extend too far out away from the bench, which also creates stress on your shoulder joints. Keep your hips close to the bench.*

TRICEPS

## DUMBBELL EXTENSION

**Starting Position:** Stand with your feet shoulder-width apart and your knees slightly bent. With both hands (palms up), grasp one end of the dumbbell behind its collar and raise it above your head.

**The Exercise:** Bending your arms, slowly lower the dumbbell behind your head. Keep your elbows close to your head and pointed straight up throughout the exercise to keep the focus on your triceps, not on your shoulders. Lower the weight until you feel a stretch in your triceps. Hold for a count of one, and press the weight back up, lifting until your arms are nearly straight and following an arc so you don't bump the back of your head.

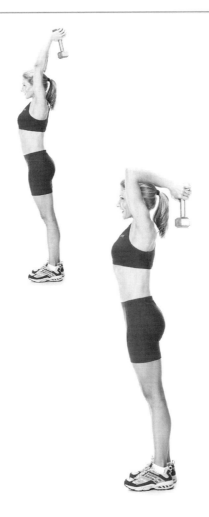

TIP

*Keep your elbows pointed up, and hold them in— don't let them flare out to the sides. Also, don't hold the dumbbell like a sandwich. Place your palms so they face the inside end plate of the dumbbell, with your index fingers and thumbs touching.*

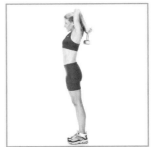

TRICEPS

## LYING DUMBBELL EXTENSION

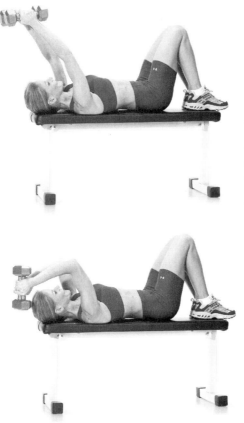

**Starting Position:** Lie down on a flat bench with a dumbbell in each hand, arms extended over your head so you are looking straight up at them, palms facing each other.

**The Exercise:** Hold the weights together. Bend your elbows and slowly lower the dumbbells toward the top of your head. Your upper arms should remain stationary. Keep your elbows pointed up, not back.

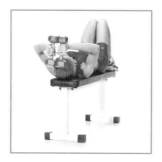

TIP

*Don't let your elbows flare out.*
*Keep them in and pointed straight up.*

TRICEPS

## TRICEPS KICKBACK

**Starting Position:** Holding a dumbbell in your left hand, stand at arm's distance from a bench, your feet hip-width apart. Resting your right palm on the surface of the bench, bend your knees slightly until your back is parallel to the floor. Tuck your left elbow close to your torso until your upper arm is parallel to the floor. Your knuckles should point toward the floor.

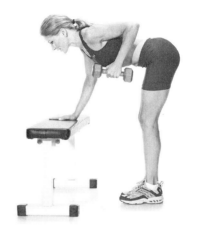

**The Exercise:** Straighten your left arm, bringing the dumbbell back and up to your hip, until your arm is fully extended and parallel to the floor (without locking your elbow). Hold; then slowly bend your elbow to the starting position. Complete your reps; then switch to your right arm.

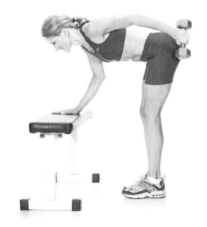

**TIP**

*Don't lift your arm too high; remember that it should be parallel to the floor. Make sure your back remains level, or parallel to the floor. Do not lift one shoulder higher than the other.*

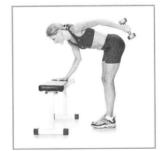

# ALTERNATING DUMBBELL CURL

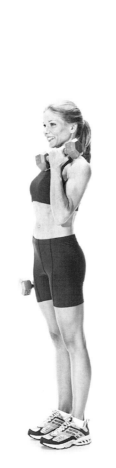

**Starting Position:** Hold a dumbbell in each hand, arms by your sides, palms facing your thighs. Stand with your feet hip-width apart, legs straight but not locked.

**The Exercise:** Keeping your torso still, bend your left elbow and bring the dumbbell up and in toward your shoulder. When you reach your shoulder, rotate your palm so that it faces inward, without allowing your elbow to move forward. Hold; then slowly lower. Alternate sides for the set. (Only one arm lifts at a time; one curl on each side equals one rep.)

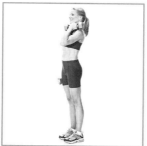

### TIP

*Don't swing your arms; keep your torso still as you do this exercise. Complete the movement with one arm before you begin with the other arm. Do not allow your elbows to move in front of your body. Keep them tucked into your side throughout the exercise. Also, your back should remain straight—do not arch your back to help lift the weights.*

## DUMBBELL CURL

**Starting Position:** Holding a dumbbell in each hand, stand with your feet hip-width apart, knees slightly bent, toes pointing in. Let your arms hang by your sides. Your elbows should be a straight line with your shoulders, and your palms should be facing forward so that your thumbs are pointing out.

**The Exercise:** Slowly bring the dumbbells up toward your shoulders. Focus on keeping your upper arms vertical and your wrists straight. Hold; then slowly lower to your starting position.

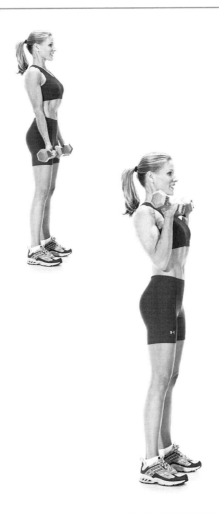

**TIP**

*Don't lean too far forward or back. Your body should be erect, which ensures that you have stability in your core. Keep your elbows tucked into your body. Do not allow them to move outward from your body.*

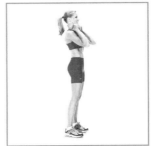

BICEPS

## SEATED DUMBBELL CURL

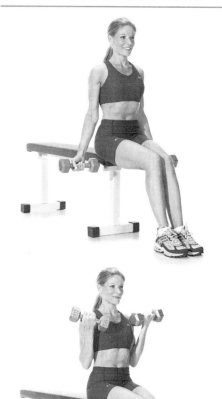

**Starting Position:** Sit on the edge of a flat bench with your arms at your sides, a dumbbell in each hand, palms facing forward.

**The Exercise:** Curl both arms, lifting the dumbbells toward your shoulders. During the curl, keep your upper arms and torso still—there will be some movement, but avoid swinging the weights up. Let your biceps do the work. Then slowly lower the dumbbells to the starting point.

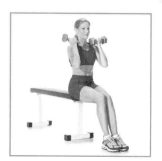

TIP

*Don't lean backward or forward as you lower the weights; doing that would cut down on the amount of work the biceps are doing.*

BICEPS

## HAMMER CURL

**Starting Position:** Stand with your feet roughly shoulder-width apart, your arms extended down at your sides, a dumbbell in each hand, and with your palms facing each other.

**The Exercise:** Curl both arms, lifting the dumbbells toward your shoulders. During the curl, keep your upper arms and torso still. Lower the dumbbells slowly back to your sides.

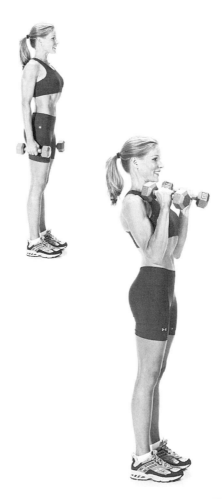

**TIP**

*Maintain straight posture throughout the exercise. Do not lean forward or backward. Keep your abs tight and your torso upright. Don't lift with your palms facing down. The proper form for lifting the dumbbells is with your palms facing each other.*

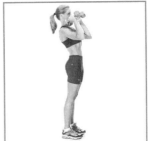

BICEPS

## DUMBBELL SQUAT

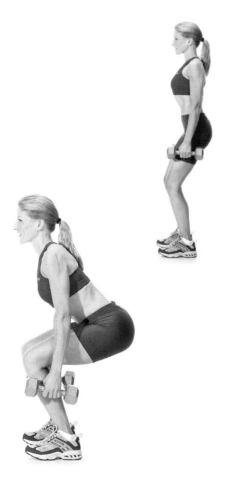

**Starting Position:** Hold two dumbbells at your sides, with your palms facing in. Stand with your feet roughly shoulder-width apart.

**The Exercise:** While keeping your shoulders, back, and head upright, bend your legs at the knees and lower your hips until your thighs are parallel with the floor. Then, pushing from your heels, lift yourself back to the starting position. Keep your back as straight as possible throughout this exercise. If you have trouble balancing, try placing a sturdy, 1-inch-thick wooden block or a couple of dumbbell plates under your heels.

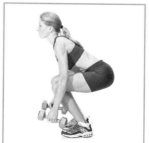

TIP

*Do not allow your knees to extend beyond your toes. Your weight should shift backward into your heels as you lower down. Keep your abdominals tight to stabilize your lower back.*

QUADRICEPS AND HAMSTRINGS

## DUMBBELL LUNGE

**Starting Position:** Stand with your feet together, toes pointed forward, a dumbbell in each hand. Keep your shoulders squared, your chin up, your back straight, and palms facing in.

**The Exercise:** Step forward with your right foot. Bend at your knees, and lower your hips until your left knee is just a few inches off the floor. Push with the right leg, raising yourself back to the starting point. Repeat until you've done the planned number of reps for your right leg; then do the same for your left leg.

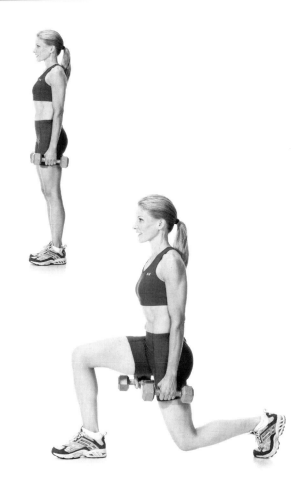

**TIP**

*Don't point your toes in or out. Both feet should point straight ahead. Also, don't lift your heel on the forward foot. Keep it flat. The proper form is with the knee on the forward leg over your ankle, not out in front of it.*

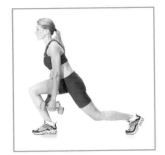

QUADRICEPS AND HAMSTRINGS

# PLIÉ DUMBBELL SQUAT

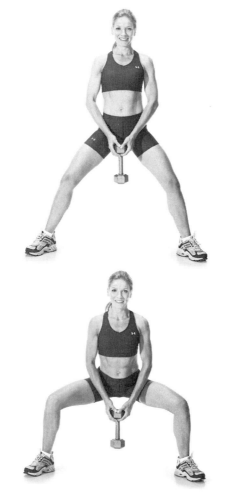

**Starting Position:** Stand with your feet about 2 to 3 feet apart, legs straight but not locked, toes pointed out at a 45-degree angle. Using both hands, hold one dumbbell vertically in front of your body, elbows slightly bent.

**The Exercise:** Move your hips back as if to sit in a chair. Then bend your knees, letting them follow the exact angle of your toes. Lower your body until your thighs are parallel with the floor. Keep your heels down and your weight evenly distributed. Return to the starting position.

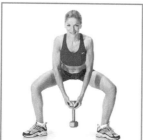

**TIP**

*Do not allow your knees to extend beyond your toes. Maintain good posture. As you perform this movement, your torso should be vertical, your chest up, and your feet flat on the ground.*

**QUADRICEPS AND HAMSTRINGS**

## STATIONARY LUNGE

**Starting Position:** Holding dumbbells at your sides, palms in, stand with your feet about 2 to 3 feet apart, your left foot in front of your right.

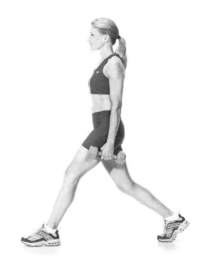

**The Exercise:** Lower your body until your front knee is bent 90 degrees and your rear knee nearly touches the floor. Your rear heel will come off the floor. Your front knee should stay behind your toes, and your torso should remain upright. Push yourself back up to the starting position. Finish all of your repetitions; then repeat the exercise with your left foot in front of your right.

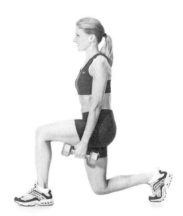

TIP

*Don't let your front knee extend beyond your toes, and keep your torso upright and your abdominals tight throughout the exercise.*

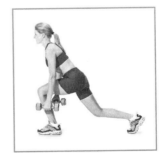

## DEADLIFT

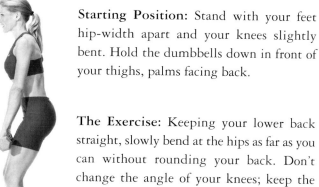

**Starting Position:** Stand with your feet hip-width apart and your knees slightly bent. Hold the dumbbells down in front of your thighs, palms facing back.

**The Exercise:** Keeping your lower back straight, slowly bend at the hips as far as you can without rounding your back. Don't change the angle of your knees; keep the dumbbells as close to your body as possible throughout. Pause; then stand back up.

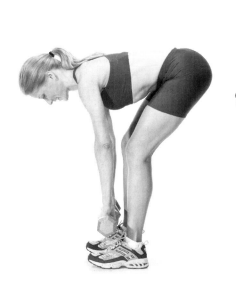

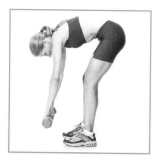

**TIP**

*Don't round your spine. If this is a problem, bend your knees a bit more and bring up your torso slightly.*

# STANDING ONE-LEG CALF RAISE

**Starting Position:** Stand with the ball of your right foot resting on a step or a sturdy wooden block, a dumbbell in your left hand, palm facing in. Holding on to something for balance with your right hand, lift your left foot and hook it behind your right calf. Lower your right heel as far as you can, really stretching your calf at the bottom.

**The Exercise:** Press up on your toes as much as possible, contracting your calf muscle. Hold that flex for a count of one; then slowly lower yourself. Repeat for the planned number of reps. Switch legs and hands (now you'll hold the weight in your right hand and hold on to the chair with your left hand), and follow the same instructions.

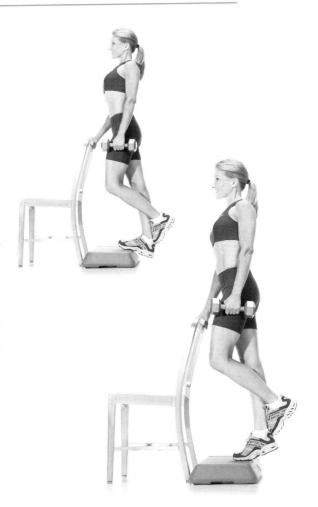

**TIP**

*Don't let your foot roll toward the little toe when you're lifting. Instead, raise yourself, flexing your calf, and put your weight on the ball of your foot. Don't lean forward, but stand up as straight as possible.*

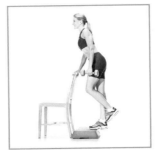

CALF

## ANGLED CALF RAISE

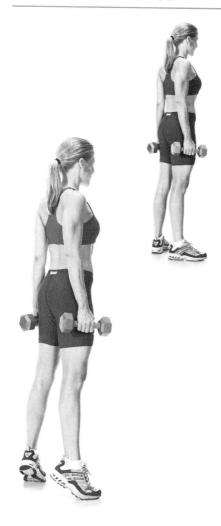

**Starting Position:** Hold a dumbbell in each hand, palms facing in, and stand with your feet about shoulder-width apart. Turn your toes out so your feet form a 45-degree angle.

**The Exercise:** Keeping your legs straight, raise yourself on your toes as high as possible. Pause for a count of one; then slowly lower yourself to the starting position.

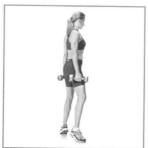

TIP

*Don't do this exercise on a carpet—find a solid surface, like a hardwood or concrete floor. Do not rotate your toes to more than a 45-degree angle because that would stress your knee joints. Also, make sure your knees are stationary and straight but not locked. Too much knee flexion inhibits calf isolation.*

CALF

# FLOOR CRUNCH

**Starting Position:** Lie on a floor (preferably a carpeted floor or a pad of some kind), put your hands beside your head, bring your knees together, and place your feet flat on the floor about a foot from your hips.

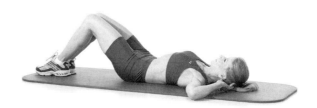

**The Exercise:** Push your lower back down, almost like you're trying to make a dent in the floor. Then begin to roll your shoulders up, keeping your knees and hips stationary. Continue to push down as hard as you can with your lower back.

When your shoulders come off the ground a few inches, hold this position and flex your abdominal muscles as hard as you can for a count of one. Then slowly lower your shoulders back down to the floor. Push down with your lower back for the entire exercise.

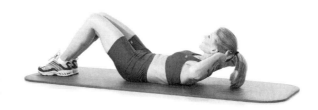

TIP

*Don't lock your hands behind your head. Your hands should be cupped at the sides of your head and should not be used for leverage.*

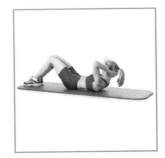

ABDOMINAL

## BALL CRUNCH

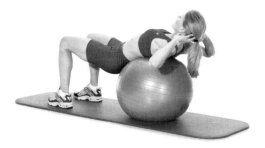

**Starting Position:** Lie on your back on an exercise ball with your hands behind your head, your feet flat on the floor, and your legs at a 90-degree angle.

**The Exercise:** Using your abs, raise your head and shoulders, and crunch your rib cage toward your pelvis. Pause; then slowly return to the starting position.

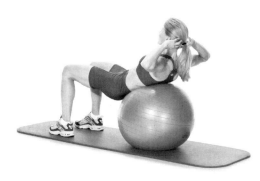

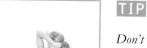

**TIP**

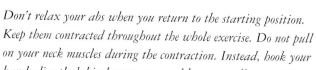

*Don't relax your abs when you return to the starting position. Keep them contracted throughout the whole exercise. Do not pull on your neck muscles during the contraction. Instead, hook your hands directly behind your ears, and keep your elbows wide. Your lower back should maintain contact with the ball.*

ABDOMINAL

# REVERSE CRUNCH

**Starting Position:** Lie on your back with your legs and hips bent at 90-degree angles, and your arms relaxed at your sides, palms facing down.

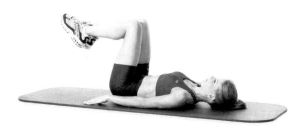

**The Exercise:** Pull your abs in, and lift your hips as if you were tipping a bucket of water that's resting on top of your pelvis.

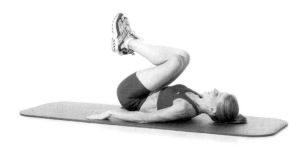

**TIP**

*Do not lift your hips to more than a 30-degree angle from the floor. Also, do not use your hands to help tilt your hips.*

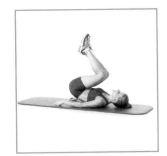

## TWIST CRUNCH

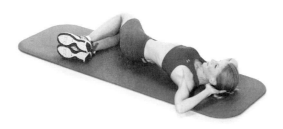

**Starting Position:** Lie flat on your back, your knees bent and your hands beside your head. Let your legs fall as far as they can to your right side so your upper body is flat on the floor and your lower body is on its side.

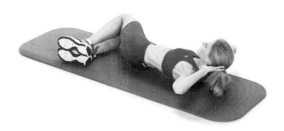

**The Exercise:** Press your lower back down into the floor while you roll your upper body slightly up until your shoulder blades clear the floor. Concentrate on your obliques (the muscles on the side of your waist), and contract and hold the crunch for a count of one. Slowly lower to the starting position. Count one, and then perform your next rep. After you complete the number of planned reps on your right side, switch to your left and follow the same instructions.

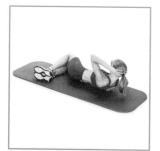

TIP

*Don't lock your hands behind your head. Don't worry how far your knees can drop to the ground. Everyone varies in flexibility. Most important, keep your shoulders square to the ceiling and contract your rib cage to your hip bones.*

ABDOMINAL

## HIP THRUST

**Starting Position:** Lie flat on your back on the floor, with your legs straight up in the air directly above your hips and your feet flexed. Stretch your arms back behind your head and grasp a leg of your bench, or any other sturdy object that can support your weight. Your shoulders should remain relaxed on the floor.

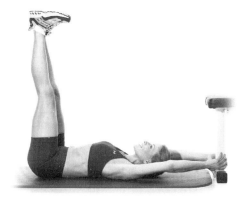

**The Exercise:** Lift with the lowest area of your abs so that your hips rise off the floor several inches. Squeeze and hold for several seconds at the top of the movement; then return to the starting position.

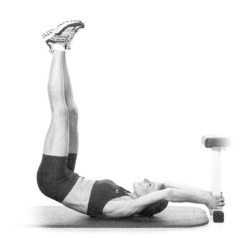

TIP

*To increase the effectiveness of this exercise, keep your legs in line with your hips.*

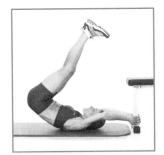

ABDOMINAL

194 • *Exercise Guide*

## SPINAL STRETCH

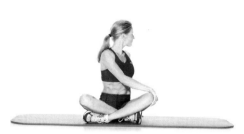

**Starting Position:** Sitting cross-legged, press your sit (derriere) bones into the floor and lengthen your spine, reaching up with the crown of your head. (If this is uncomfortable, sit on a firm pillow or folded blanket, or extend one leg.) Keep both sit bones on the floor while you do this stretch.

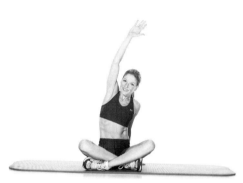

**The Exercise:** (a) Place your right hand on your left knee, inhale, and lengthen your spine. Then exhale and twist to the left. Breathe, return to center, switch sides, and repeat. (b) Place your left hand on the floor, close to your body, and extend your right arm overhead. Inhale and reach your fingers toward the ceiling, stretching your right side. Then exhale and reach to the left, stretching your left side. Switch sides and repeat.

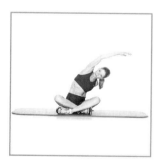

TIP

*If your left sit bone comes off the floor, don't stretch so far. Breathe, switch sides, and repeat, reaching to the left.*

STRETCHES

## CAT TILT

**Starting Position:** Get on all fours, with your wrists under your shoulders, and your knees under your hips. Lengthen your spine, reaching the crown of your head toward the wall in front of you and your tailbone toward the wall behind you. Inhale deeply, then exhale and round your back toward the ceiling like an angry cat, drawing your chin toward your navel.

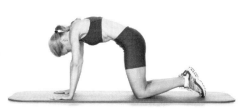

**The Exercise:** On the next inhale, arch your back, dropping your belly toward the floor, lifting your sit bones and collarbones, and gazing toward the ceiling. Repeat this sequence three times.

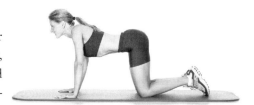

TIP

*Do not hyperextend your neck when you're arching your back; instead, tuck your head downward and in toward your abdomen.*

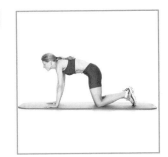

STRETCHES

## PUPPY DOG

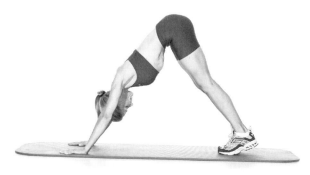

**Starting Position:** From all fours, (a) press your hands and fingers into the floor, and (b) raise your knees, lifting your hips up and back, until you are in an upside-down V.

**The Exercise:** Keeping both knees slightly bent and your head in line with your back, breathe and push your shoulders slightly through your arms, toward the floor. Release one knee and try to push the opposite heel to the floor. Then reverse.

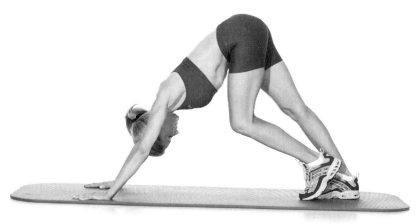

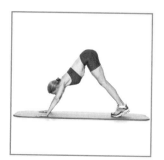

**TIP**

*Do not bounce. Bend only one knee at a time, and keep the movements slow and controlled to allow the muscles to relax. Do not raise your head, but keep it in line with your back.*

## LUNGE

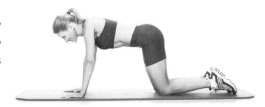

**Starting Position:** Get on all fours. Step your right foot forward so your toes line up with your fingers, and your front knee is over your ankle.

**The Exercise:** Next, slide your left leg behind you with your knee on the floor. Keep your spine long and straight and your shoulder blades down. Breathe, switch sides, and repeat.

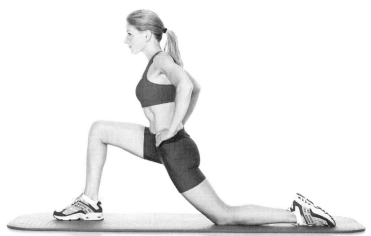

TIP

*To deepen the stretch, press your hips forward and down and your collarbones up. Do not allow your front knee to extend beyond your ankle.*

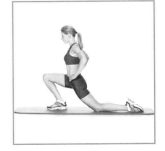

STRETCHES

## RUNNER'S STRETCH

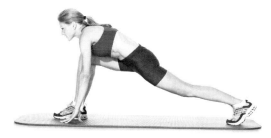

**Starting Position:** From the Lunge, lift your hips toward the ceiling, sliding your hands back a little and letting your front leg straighten as much as possible.

**The Exercise:** Press your back heel toward the floor, allowing your toes to angle out slightly. Keeping your legs as straight as possible, with hips reaching toward the ceiling, relax your upper body down over your front thigh. Breathe; then switch sides and repeat.

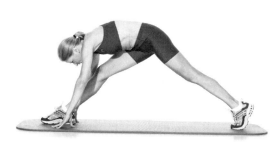

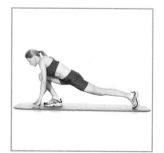

TIP

*Do not allow your knee to extend forward over your toes or beyond. If you are not flexible enough to put your hands on the floor, place a bench next to you to help you to keep your balance.*

# TRIANGLE POSE

**Starting Position:** From the Runner's Stretch, with your right leg forward, place your right hand on your right shin or ankle, and your left hand on your left hip. Turn your left foot so your toes point to the left; right toes point forward.

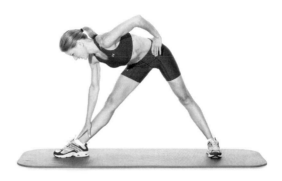

**The Exercise:** Roll your torso open to the left so your left shoulder lines up over your right shoulder. (If you feel steady, lift your left arm straight toward the ceiling so it's in line with your right arm. Keep your spine long, and look up at your left arm. If this bothers your neck, gaze straight ahead.) Breathe; then switch sides and repeat.

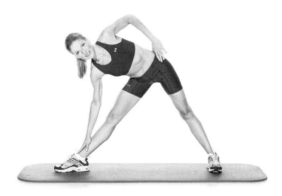

TIP

*Only twist if you feel comfortable. If you are fairly inflexible, start with just the Runner's Stretch, and build up to the Triangle Pose. Do not twist too far—your shoulders should stack on top of each other to maintain proper alignment.*

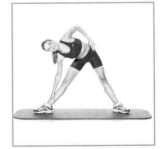

STRETCHES

# Questions and Answers

## Appendix B

Q: *The only time I can do my daily workout is 6:00 A.M., before work. I want to get on the treadmill, but I just can't make it out of bed. I think, "It's too cold, too dark, too early." I know I should do it, I say I should do it, but most mornings, I don't. Then I feel guilty for the rest of the day. Why can't I get it together?*

A: Hmm. It sounds like you *are* hopping on the treadmill each morning—the coulda/shoulda/woulda treadmill. That treadmill will get you nowhere fast.

I don't always like dragging myself out of bed at 5:00 or 6:00 A.M. for my workout, either, but I do it anyway. Why? Because exercise is a gift that I give myself—the gift of health and vitality. On those I-don't-wanna days, I have a mind-over-mattress dialogue with myself. Try it. When you wake up, open your eyes, and start hearing the excuses, say to yourself, "It's not too dark or too early to give myself the gift of a fit, healthy body."

So, as hard as it is, hop out of bed, slide into your sweats, and get to it. By now, you should have come up with a Target Motivation Mantra (if you haven't, see part 3 on how to develop one). Say it over and over again to stay focused on your goal and to give yourself the extra oomph you need to get out of bed each morning. If you can get yourself out of bed for just a few consecutive days, you're likely to find that it becomes much easier—and that you're actually enjoying this time to yourself.

Q: *I'm 35 years old, and I have 50 pounds to lose. I'm following the program, but the weight is coming off so slowly! I've tried virtually every diet known to woman, and I'm scared that I've wrecked my metabolism. What's going on?*

A: It's true that years of crash-and-starvation dieting can significantly reduce a woman's basal metabolic rate (BMR). But don't panic—you can definitely rev it up again.

Metabolism is based on genetics, thyroid function, and muscle mass. Assuming that your thyroid is fine, the Body-*for*-LIFE for Women Training Method will build calorie-burning muscle, and the Body-*for*-LIFE for Women Eating Method will give you the fuel you need for building that muscle, nourishing your body, and keeping food cravings at bay. Over time, as you train and eat smart, your body fat—along with your total body weight—will start to fall. The key is to be patient as your body adapts to the healthier Body-*for*-LIFE lifestyle.

One more thing: Remember, you don't have 50 pounds to "lose"; you have 50 pounds to *remove*. Losing anything means you want to find it again. Not so, that extra body fat, right? On fad diets, you lose and find the same excess body fat. On Body-*for*-LIFE for Women, you'll remove it once and for all.

Q: *What should I do after 12 weeks?*

A: That depends on the amount of weight you want to remove. If you have less than 20 pounds to remove, you may find that you've reached your goal by the end of Segment 1. Then you can move straight into Maintenance. You may want to use the Alternate Weight Maintenance Formula (see Appendix D) to adjust your caloric intake and physical-activity requirements to your new, fitter body.

If you have more than 20 pounds to remove, then you'll repeat the Segments until you achieve your goal weight. Then you'll move to Maintenance. But with each Segment—and even into Maintenance—you'll continue to set new goals and move forward.

Regardless of how much weight you wish to remove, keep the focus on developing your mental outlook, along with your body. That's a critical component to the success of this program. I've seen hundreds of women, in 12 short weeks, become more self-confident, more willing to fight for their right to self-care, and more ready to take on new challenges, physical or otherwise. They also develop new, *lasting* healthy patterns—following the Body-*for*-LIFE for Women Eating Method, continuing to challenge themselves in their weight training and cardio, and using the Power Mind Principles to fight stress, achieve balance in their lives, and stay on track.

It doesn't matter how long it takes you to reach your goal weight. It's the journey that's important. Your mind will keep your body fit. And you never really leave the program—it's always there for you. The ultimate goal is to *sustain* whatever you have achieved and to regroup immediately if you slip.

Q: *I'm 40 and need to shed about 70 pounds. I have high cholesterol, and my blood sugar is borderline high. How fast can I shed the weight and reverse these medical problems?*

A: If you stick with the program, you can expect to remove about 25 pounds during Segment 1. However, if you regularly starved yourself thin in your teens, twenties, and thirties, or gained and lost the same body fat over and over again, your metabolism may need a period of readjustment before it kicks into high gear.

Don't worry too much about how fast you'll lose—you're not in a race. I'm betting that by the end of Segment 1, you'll already be fitter—and healthier. To me, that's progress—significant progress.

Please don't allow your eagerness to get healthy to cause you to attempt to remove more than about 2 or 3 pounds of body fat per week. That's a weekly caloric deficit of 7,000 to 10,500 calories. Losing more than that can cause you to lose muscle, which is not good. Remember, the more muscle you have, the more calories you burn. You definitely don't want to lose muscle—your metabolism could sputter, putting an end to your fat loss.

Remember that your goal is to lose fat, not just "weight." So I recommend that you test your body fat after each Segment to track your progress. You can buy a device called skin-fold calipers, buy a scale that calculates body fat, or go to almost any local gym and have it tested.

Q: *I have seen the pictures of women in the original Body-for-LIFE book. They look so muscular and sculpted. Is that supposed to be my goal? I just want to feel healthier, have more energy, and feel better about myself.*

A: The pictures in the first *Body-for-LIFE* reflect the accomplishments of women whose goal was to achieve that specific look. Indeed, all of the women featured in this book (and on the covers) have also achieved amazing results, which was a reward they earned for sticking faithfully to the eating plan, continually ramping up their training intensity, and honoring their commitments to themselves. These women worked very hard to achieve that visual goal because it was important to them. You can see that in this book, we included what we call "after-after" photos, of women who've sustained their results for many years on the Body-*for*-LIFE plan. As a doctor, it pleases me to know that for the majority of women, especially those 40 and older, health—not abs—is the driving motivation. Your goals are right on, girlfriend. If you drop your BMI, body fat percentage, waist circumference, and total body weight into the healthy range, you will achieve all of your goals—and more.

Q: *I'm 4 weeks into Segment 2, and I've hit a plateau. This always happens to me, and it's so frustrating. What am I doing wrong?*

A: Probably nothing. Your age, body composition, and metabolism (some women have a hotter "furnace" than others) all play a role in how quickly you will remove weight. But you may also need to readjust your training or eating regimen.

This is where your Mind-Mouth-Muscle Daily Journals come in. Review them (if you're not keeping them, I urge you to start). If you've removed some weight and then stopped, have you updated your Weight Removal Formula (see Appendix D) and made the appropriate readjustments in your caloric intake and physical activity? This can be useful, because an extra 200 calories a day can amount to a 20-pound weight gain in 1 year. Have you watched your portion sizes and kept to Smart Proteins, Carbs, and Fats? Or have Junk Carbs crept back into your daily eating? Have you turned to food again to relieve stress, instead of following the Power Mind Principles?

If you're following the program exactly, try increasing the intensity and frequency of your workouts. For example, if you're doing cardio four times a week, increase it to five. It may be that after 4 weeks, your body has adapted to the stress of your current cardio and weight training, so the total number of calories you burn has decreased. Your muscles don't have to work as hard, so your energy expenditure has decreased. Cross-training will challenge your body as well.

After you try all this, wait and watch. Sometimes it takes several weeks to bust a plateau. Odds are, your patience and persistence will pay off.

Q: *I'm following the program but am having a very hard time fighting my need to do it perfectly. I've messed up a few times—just a little bit. Each time, I figured that I'd blown it, so I spent the rest of the day overeating and beating myself up. How can I stop doing this?*

A: So you had a cookie (or five) at the office, or a few more chips (okay, half a bag) than you would have liked. It's okay. Really, it is. So please, please, *please*, stop beating yourself up. Not only is your self-abuse ineffective; it's ultimately self-destructive. If you continue to punish yourself for each little slip, sooner or later you'll go off the program altogether. I don't want that, and I'm betting you don't, either.

I recommend that you focus on Power Mind Principle 5: Aim for progress, not perfection. I'm sure it will be hard for you to follow, but it's extremely important that you try. You can't change your body, or a less-than-healthy lifestyle, overnight. All you can do is your best.

You should also adopt the Rule of Reverse Expectations, which means that you should plan on making mistakes. We all do! Remember, all you really need to do is follow the program 80 percent of the time. The other 20 percent of the time, you get to be imperfect. Give yourself permission to mess up. You'll find that being loving to yourself gets you closer to your goals than does nasty, negative self-talk.

Q: *My husband wants to do Body-for-LIFE together. I've agreed, but I'm dreading it because he always drops weight much more quickly than I do. I get so resentful and depressed that I give up and it affects our relationship. How can we work together?*

A: It's great that your partner wants to team up with you. I'd say you're lucky! But I also see your point—when it comes to weight removal, men do seem to have it easier.

There are several reasons for this. First, the average man has more muscle mass than the average woman does, which gives him a higher basal metabolic rate. Thus, he's able to burn calories faster than a woman can. And because men are just plain bigger than women, they can eat more than we can without gaining weight, and they can build muscle faster because of their male sex hormones and testosterone.

I recommend that you support his efforts, as he's sure to support yours. It will also be helpful to get your expectations squared away before you start. Accept that he will remove body fat faster than you do. Expect it. And no matter how tempted you are, don't ask him how much weight he's removed. In fact, ask him not to share that information with you. This program isn't just about numbers—you're learning to care for yourself.

Continue to support each other, but work out at your own pace. If he wants to go harder or faster, let him. Eat according to *your* caloric needs. He may build muscle and burn fat faster than you, but if you follow this program, you will, too—guaranteed.

Q: *I can follow the Body-for-LIFE for Women Eating Method plan with no problems—I'm never hungry, and I've learned to put together delicious meals from the Smart Foods table. But it all goes to pot the week before my period, when I crave sweets—chocolate, cookies, and especially ice cream. I try to resist, but it's hard not to polish off a pint of ice cream when I'm moody and bloated. Help!*

A: I totally relate—PMS tests the resolve of the strongest women. I'm not immune to the PMS munchies; I just have to have my jelly beans. Here's the thing, though: Because you know you have cravings for sweets a week before your period, why not plan for them so you can minimize the damage?

To discourage cravings, make sure to eat every few hours, have a bit of protein at every meal, and eliminate foods made with white sugar and white flour, like white bread, pasta, and rice. These Junk Carbs will cause your blood sugar to soar, then plummet, which will trigger even more cravings for junk. To keep bloat under control, limit your intake of whole grains and starches to no more than two or three servings per day, and eat them before 5:00 P.M. When you need a sweet, have a bowl of mixed berries and fresh ricotta cheese. You also might want to check out the *Eating-for-LIFE* cookbook. It contains tons of healthy desserts that only taste decadent. Plan to have one or two over the course of this week. This tip might be especially helpful if you know that when you eat refined sugar, you tend to binge.

I know what you're thinking: What if I do all that and I still want the ice cream? Then eat it. To tell a moody, bloated woman that she can't have a cup of ice cream would make me a traitor to my gender. Just be smart about it. Have one serving, savor it, and try to get back on the program the next day.

Q: *Like many women, I overeat when I'm stressed. The problem is, I'm stressed every day, with work, my family, and other obligations. I try to control myself, but food is so soothing. Is there hope for me?*

A: Before I answer your question, I want you to answer this one: If your best friend asked you the question you just asked me, what would you say?

Most likely, you'd say that you understood—that you eat under stress, too. But you might also say that she needed to deal with her stress in a positive way—take some time for herself, splurge on a nonfood treat. No matter what your exact words, I'm pretty sure you would tell her that she owes it to herself to manage her stress before it wrecks her physical health and quality of life.

Well, that's what I'm telling you. As stressed-out as your life is, it will be less stressed-out if you learn to become your own caretaker and deal with stress in constructive ways, rather than in ways that hurt you.

I suggest that you reread part 3. When you're done, pick two tools that you then commit to trying before you head for food. Many of my female patients have told me that they posted the Stress Rx signs (pages 77 to 78) in the appropriate places *before* stress hit them, and they found that seeing the signs posted on the refrigerator door, or on their treadmill or gym bag, helped them immensely.

Of course, there are practical things you can do to short-circuit stress eating. For one thing, make sure you eat every few hours so that you're not actually hungry. When you feel those stress-fueled cravings coming on, turn to the Smart Proteins and Smart Carbs—say, two pieces of low-fat string cheese and a piece of fruit. Finally, whether you're at home or the office, take a short walk, even if it's just up and down the stairwell a few times. Physical activity increases your endorphins, which dampen the stress response and leave you feeling calmer and in control.

Don't give up. This program is all about growth and reaching beyond perceived limitations. Believe it or not, you can conquer stress. You just have to take care of yourself the way you'd care for your child or best friend.

*Q: My 18-year-old daughter and I have teamed up to do the program. We each want to remove about 20 pounds. I'm 45 and put on my weight in my forties. She's been heavy since she entered her teens. What can we accomplish in the first 12 weeks?*

A: How great that you and your daughter are working together! This program gives women of all generations the opportunity to join together to get physically and mentally fit.

Because your daughter is in Milestone 1, she'll probably remove weight a bit faster than you will, being in Milestone 3. But you never know—she may struggle and need you more than you expected. Whatever happens, don't compare your progress with hers. Just support her, and lean on her when you need support.

A word about removing weight quickly: Body-*for*-LIFE for Women isn't a quick fix; it's a way of life. Though all women want to remove weight yesterday, it's the women who remove it at a slow, steady rate who keep it off. Why? Because they take that time to develop and practice healthy habits that stick. If it takes you 6 months to remove 20 pounds, and you keep it off, so what? That's preferable to dumping 20 pounds in a month, returning to the habits that caused your weight gain in the first place, and regaining the weight and then some.

You and your daughter are lucky—each of you will be the other's cheerleader and help encourage healthy habits.

Q: *After years of dieting misery, I made the decision never to step on a scale again. Looking at the number on the scale upsets me. I don't even want to use a scale that measures body fat. Do I have to weigh myself?*

A: Your scale phobia is quite common among my female patients. And of course you don't have to weigh yourself. Body-*for*-LIFE for Women isn't about the number on the scale, anyway. It's about developing mental and physical power, being healthy and happy, and living up to your potential. So by all means, bag the scale if you want to.

Instead of using the scale to track your progress, choose a piece of clothing—a pair of jeans, maybe—that you really like and can get into right now but can't completely zip or button. Say you're a comfortable size 16. Either use your tightest size 16 jeans or, if 16s are baggy, take a size 14 and use that. Hang them outside your closet so that you see them when you get up and before bed. It's a visual reminder to keep focused on your Body-*for*-LIFE goals. Once a week, try 'em on. If they're looser, you're removing excess body fat. It's that simple. If they're tighter, of course, it's time to reassess.

Q: *At 60, I've spent most of my life being inactive. I want to try the program, but maybe it's simply too late for me to get in shape.*

A: It's *never* too late. Research clearly has shown that women of any age—even women in their nineties—can achieve significant improvements in body composition, strength, endurance, and flexibility.

So come on—start the program today. Your first step: Schedule an appointment with your doctor and bring this book with you. After you get a clean bill of health, ask if this program is right for you. Your doctor will work with you to suggest any tweaking to account for your health, fitness level, and age. I'd also suggest that you scout around for local health clubs or community centers for weight training and cardio classes geared to women who are at least 60 years old. The trainers who run these programs have experience working with older women, and they can teach you how to adapt this program to your needs.

At 60, you're likely to find that it will take time to remove body fat and build muscle. Again, be patient and persistent. Every step you take on the treadmill or the walking path, and every minute spent lifting weights, brings you one step closer to your ultimate goal: to get and stay healthy, fit, and vital.

Q: *My daughter is 16, and in the past few years, she's really put on weight. She's become depressed and withdrawn, which has affected her social life. I need to shed weight and get fit. I plan to start your program. Would it be appropriate for her?*

A: First, I applaud you for recognizing that your daughter is on a path that is affecting her physical and emotional well-being now and could impact it into adulthood. Kudos to you, too, for getting your own self-care together. This program is fine for young women who are 16 and over.

Approach your daughter gently. You might casually mention that you'll be starting the program and ask her if she'd like to join you. If she says no, don't push—simply start the program without her. By quietly practicing what you preach, she'll see changes in you that may motivate her to join you. The key is to get her to see that eating well and getting more active can boost her mood as well as her sense of self-esteem.

If, happily, she says yes, she can follow the entire program. Encourage her to limit or eliminate teen favorites that pack on the pounds—Junk Carbs like chips, soda, candy, and doughnuts. Instead, encourage her to eat Smart Foods—lots of fruits and veggies, fish, poultry, whole grains—and make sure she gets her iron and calcium.

Q: *As you recommend, I'm adding more intensity to my cardio workouts. I walk outside and have added hills as well as speed to get the sweat going. However, I don't belong to a gym and would prefer to do the strength training at home. Is that okay?*

A: You bet. In fact, when I put together the training routine, I assumed that some women would want to do the workout at home. You can assemble a beginners' home gym with one set of adjustable dumbbells, an adjustable exercise bench, and a padded mat.

If you'd rather get single-poundage dumbbells, that's fine, too. You can stow them out of sight easily in a closet or under the bed. They're also versatile. Use free weights along with benches or Swiss balls, and you'll have a multitude of exercise options.

Q: *I have a bad problem with eating at night. I follow the program all day—until 8:00 P.M. By 11:00, I've eaten an extra 600 or 700 calories. I can't seem to help myself—I feel so hungry! Any suggestions?*

A: Are you eating small, nutritious meals five to six times a day, including a midafternoon snack and a reasonable after-dinner snack about 90 minutes before bed? If so, then I suspect the problem isn't that you're hungry. It's that you want to eat.

Hunger is a physical need for food—your stomach growls, and you may feel weak or light-headed. By contrast, appetite is a psychological need for food. Appetite is when you walk past a bakery and want a doughnut, despite the fact that you just had a satisfying lunch.

Understand that you've gotten into the habit of eating at night, and what you think is hunger is simply the habit of eating when you want food, not when you need it. There's lots you can do to break that habit. Call upon your support system. Take a bath. Get to bed earlier; sometimes, the night munchies signal that it's sleep you need, rather than food. If you can stick it out for 3 days without eating at night, you're golden. You can do it!

Q: *I'm disgusted and depressed with the 15 pounds I've gained since I turned 40. I have constant fatigue, bloating, chocolate cravings, and mood swings, which are especially bad before my period. My cycle is irregular, my waist is gone, my breasts are bigger— even my back is fat. What can this program do for me?*

A: Welcome to Milestone 3, which is where I am right now. As a physician, I know that women in this milestone are more prone to depression and mood shifts, especially when their sex hormones are in flux. You're experiencing the double whammy of premenstrual moodiness and the beginning of estrogen withdrawal, which can have a significant effect on a woman's menstrual cycle and moods.

As a woman, I know how lousy it can feel to have your body change before your very eyes. Integrating the Mind-Mouth-Muscle Formula into your life will definitely help ease perimenopausal symptoms. Learning techniques that can help you navigate the stress of these body changes, eating well, and moving your body regularly will dampen the urge to succumb to dark moods and overeating.

Above all, remember that the women who have the fittest bodies—and minds—struggle less with the physical and mental changes of perimenopause. On the Body-*for*-LIFE program, either you will remove excess body fat if you need to, or you will stabilize your weight so that you don't gain more. Plus, you'll be healthy and fit. Any way you look at it, you're a winner. If, however, you've done what you can to optimize your lifestyle, and your symptoms are still unbearable, ask your doctor about the appropriate therapies that can bring you relief in the short term.

Q: *My doctor recently diagnosed me with hypothyroidism and put me on thyroid medication. However, I'd already gained 30 pounds by the time he figured out what was wrong, and even with the medication, the extra weight won't come off. Help!*

A: Autoimmune conditions like hypothyroidism are very common in women. Unfortunately, so are the symptoms, including weight gain and increased body fat. The good news is that you can remove the weight.

This kind of weight gain can be removed by stepping up the intensity of physical activity. Are you doing your cardio five times a week? Try adding a sixth day, and make sure that you're working at the highest intensity that's comfortable for you. You'll also want to pay special attention to how much you're eating. You can't trust your instincts on this, because they have been confused by a lower-than-normal thyroid hormone level.

Removing the 30 pounds will probably take two 12-week Segments. You may reach your goal before the end of the second Segment. If so, then shift to the Weight Maintenance Formula and begin to practice your weight maintenance.

Q: *I've just had a hysterectomy. I've been placed on hormone therapy (estrogen only) to help alleviate the symptoms of surgical menopause, but I'm worried about gaining a lot of weight in a short period of time. Will the program help me avoid this?*

A: When women enter menopause, they tend to accumulate fat on their upper bodies. However, in natural menopause, that fat gain is gradual. Women who enter menopause because of surgery or medications may gain it in a shorter period of time.

But—and this is an important *but*—if you are on a low-dose hormonal replacement and you're following the Body-*for*-LIFE for Women program, most likely you won't gain any more weight than the average woman in menopause. The plan will help you minimize that body fat and will provide the tools you need in order to be as firm and as fit as you can be during this stage of your life.

Q: *I'm 38 and plan to get pregnant this year. I'm excited, but I'm also worried about not losing the weight after I deliver. I have a family history of obesity, and I'm already 20 pounds overweight. Any suggestions on how to get the extra fat off now—and later?*

A: Congratulations on your decision to start your family! Although obesity runs in your family and you may have to work harder than other women to maintain a healthy weight, Body-*for*-LIFE for Women should benefit both you and your baby, even before you become pregnant.

First, make plans to start Segment 1 of the Body-*for*-LIFE for Women Training Method. If you stick to the program and there are no extenuating circumstances, you should be able to remove those 20 pounds. When you reach your goal weight, go straight into Maintenance to cement your new body composition and lifestyle habits. Then you're off and running.

When you get pregnant, tell your doctor about your program—what you're eating, how often you train—and keep him informed throughout your pregnancy so he can adjust your diet and physical activity. If you gain a healthy amount of pregnancy weight (20 to 35 pounds), you'll be able to remove it by 4 to 6 months after you deliver.

Q: *I truly believe that I'm addicted to sugar. Every time I try to have just one cookie, I end up polishing off the whole box. My sugar binges have gotten even worse since I stopped smoking a few months ago. My mother, who was an alcoholic, had a worse sweet tooth than mine. Is it possible to be addicted to sugar?*

A: Yes. Recent studies have shown that a craving for sweets may stem from an "addiction gene" that controls addictive behaviors like alcoholism. So a love for sweets may be a marker of addiction. What's more, women who carry the gene but who are *not* addicted to alcohol or tobacco can be "addicted" to sugar.

The fact that you are an ex-smoker whose sugar cravings got worse when you quit is telling; many former smokers and alcoholics in recovery shift their addiction to sugar. Most are unaware that when they eat sugar, they are actually "smoking" or "drinking" that sugary food in front of them. One of my sugar-addicted patients had a grandmother who was an alcoholic. She was able to fight her craving for alcohol by envisioning herself "drinking" her favorite cookies or candy. Talk about effective!

However, most women who are addicted to sugar know it. My advice is to do your best to avoid all refined and processed sugars. It's important to know that eating a serving of Smart Protein, like a piece of low-fat string cheese, can curb sugar cravings significantly. Also, learn how to satisfy your sweet tooth with one or all of the following substitutes: fruit (opt for water-filled fruits, such as apples and berries, and avoid fruits that contain a lot of sugar, such as grapes and bananas); sucralose (Splenda); fructose; or the herb stevia.

# Daily Progress Reports

*Appendix C*

*Body-for-LIFE for Women*                    *Mind-Mouth-Muscle Daily Journal: Mind*

| Date: | Day _____ of 84 |
|---|---|

The Rule of Reverse Expectations: Approach any and all obstacles in your path not as problems, but as opportunities to learn to stay the course with your self-care.

### DAILY REGROUPING REPORT

If your plan A gets off track today . . .

What happened, and how did you get your eating and/or training back on track?

### DAILY STRESS REPORT

If you had a stressful day . . .

What happened: Did you deal with the stress in a positive way ("The answer is here") or in a negative way ("The answer is not here")?

Did you take recovery time throughout the day? Did you do your relaxation technique?

### DAILY JOY REPORT

My Daily Joy was:

*If you didn't joy yourself today, please do it tomorrow!*

### DAILY GRATITUDE REPORT

What are you grateful for in your life today?

*Body-for-LIFE for Women*                    *Mind-Mouth-Muscle Daily Journal: Mouth*

| Date: | Day _____ of 84 |
|---|---|

| Total portions of Smart Protein: | Total portions of Smart Protein: |
|---|---|
| Total portions of Smart Carbs: | Total portions of Smart Carbs: |
| Total portions of Smart Fats: | Total portions of Smart Fats: |

| PLAN | ACTUAL |
|---|---|
| MEAL 1 ☐ A.M. ☐ P.M. | MEAL 1 ☐ A.M. ☐ P.M. |
| MEAL 2 ☐ A.M. ☐ P.M. | MEAL 2 ☐ A.M. ☐ P.M. |
| MEAL 3 ☐ A.M. ☐ P.M. | MEAL 3 ☐ A.M. ☐ P.M. |
| MEAL 4 ☐ A.M. ☐ P.M. | MEAL 4 ☐ A.M. ☐ P.M. |
| MEAL 5 ☐ A.M. ☐ P.M. | MEAL 5 ☐ A.M. ☐ P.M. |
| MEAL 6 ☐ A.M. ☐ P.M. | MEAL 6 ☐ A.M. ☐ P.M. |

*Veggies* ☐ ☐ ☐ ☐

*Calcium-rich foods* ☐ ☐ ☐

*Water* ☐ ☐ ☐ ☐ ☐ ☐ ☐ ☐ ☐ ☐

*Mini Chill* ☐

HOW DID YOU DO?

_____

_____

_____

*Body*-for-LIFE *for Women*                    *Mind-Mouth-Muscle Daily Journal: Muscle*

| Date: | Planned Start Time: | Actual Start Time: |
|---|---|---|
| Day _____ of 84 | Planned End Time: | Actual End Time: |
| *Cardio* | Time to Complete: | Total Time: |

| Exercises Performed | PLAN | | | | ACTUAL | | | |
|---|---|---|---|---|---|---|---|---|
| | How Long? | Where | With Whom? | Intensity Level | How Long? | Where | With Whom? | Intensity Level |
| | | | | | | | | |
| | | | | | | | | |
| | | | | | | | | |

HOW DID YOU DO?

_____

_____

_____

*Body-for-LIFE for Women*                    *Mind-Mouth-Muscle Daily Journal: Muscle*

| Date: | Planned Start Time: | Actual Start Time: |
|---|---|---|
| Day _____ of 84 | Planned End Time: | Actual End Time: |
| *Upper-Body Workout* | Time to Complete: | Total Time: |

| | | PLAN | | | | | ACTUAL | | | | |
|---|---|---|---|---|---|---|---|---|---|---|---|
| Muscle Group | Exercises Performed | Sets | Reps | Weight (lb) | Minutes Between Sets | Intensity Level | Sets | Reps | Weight (lb) | Minutes Between Sets | Intensity Level |
| Chest | | | | | | | | | | | |
| | | | | | | | | | | | |
| | | | | | | | | | | | |
| Shoulders | | | | | | | | | | | |
| | | | | | | | | | | | |
| | | | | | | | | | | | |
| Back | | | | | | | | | | | |
| | | | | | | | | | | | |
| | | | | | | | | | | | |
| Triceps | | | | | | | | | | | |
| | | | | | | | | | | | |
| | | | | | | | | | | | |
| Biceps | | | | | | | | | | | |
| | | | | | | | | | | | |
| | | | | | | | | | | | |

HOW DID YOU DO?

*Body*-for-LIFE *for Women*                    *Mind-Mouth-Muscle Daily Journal: Muscle*

| Date: | Planned Start Time: | Actual Start Time: |
|---|---|---|
| Day _____ of 84 | Planned End Time: | Actual End Time: |
| *Lower-Body Workout* | Time to Complete: | Total Time: |

| Muscle Group | Exercises Performed | PLAN | | | | | ACTUAL | | | | |
|---|---|---|---|---|---|---|---|---|---|---|---|
| | | Sets | Reps | Weight (lb) | Minutes Between Sets | Intensity Level | Sets | Reps | Weight (lb) | Minutes Between Sets | Intensity Level |
| Quadriceps and Hamstrings | | | | | | | | | | | |
| | | | | | | | | | | | |
| | | | | | | | | | | | |
| Calves | | | | | | | | | | | |
| | | | | | | | | | | | |
| | | | | | | | | | | | |
| Abs | | | | | | | | | | | |
| | | | | | | | | | | | |
| | | | | | | | | | | | |

HOW DID YOU DO?

_____

_____

_____

_____

*Body-for-LIFE for Women*                    *Mind-Mouth-Muscle Daily Journal: Muscle*

| Date: | Planned Start Time: | Actual Start Time: |
|---|---|---|
| Day _____ of 84 | Planned End Time: | Actual End Time: |
| *Stretches* | Time to Complete: | Total Time: |

| Exercises | PLAN | | ACTUAL | |
|---|---|---|---|---|
| | Performed? | Length of Time Stretched | Performed? | Length of Time Stretched |
| Spinal Stretch | ☐ | | ☐ | |
| Cat Tilt | ☐ | | ☐ | |
| Puppy Dog | ☐ | | ☐ | |
| Lunge | ☐ | | ☐ | |
| Runner's Stretch | ☐ | | ☐ | |
| Triangle Pose | ☐ | | ☐ | |

HOW DID YOU DO?

_____

_____

_____

_____

# Alternate Options and Formulas

*Appendix D*

## Alternate Portion-Monitoring Options

Some women hate counting calories; some feel like they're in a dietary free fall without the safety net of close monitoring. The beauty is, the Body-*for*-LIFE for Women Eating Method can accommodate all of our individual caloric idiosyncrasies. Here are your options.

**Option 1: Paring Portions.** This option works best if you practice portion control more often than not, are conscious of the general calorie density of the foods you eat, know when you tend to overeat (sitting in front of the tube, for example), and tend to be more of a mindless eater than an emotional eater. This option may also resonate if you're beginning your first Weight Removal Segment and have at least 20 pounds to remove, and simply want to concentrate on eliminating junk foods, cutting portions of all foods, eating Smart Foods, and getting the ball rolling with your weight removal. You can actually reach your Body-*for*-LIFE for Women goal with Option 1 alone.

**Option 2: Paring Portions with Minimal Caloric Monitoring.** This option works best for women who, in addition to paring portions, need a bit more caloric monitoring to increase their awareness of subtle overeating. You might begin to check labels and keep tabs on calories as they accumulate through the day. Option 2 women include those who eat mindlessly or emotionally, have that last 10 to 15 pounds to remove and are fine-tuning their eating to achieve their goal, or are so close to achieving their goal weight that every calorie counts (or have achieved their goal weight and now need to maintain it). Finally, women who've reached goal weight and are starting the Weight Maintenance Segments may benefit from a quick calorie check-in to become more aware of their new calorie allowance.

**Option 3: Paring Portions with More-Focused Caloric Monitoring.** Rather than "checking in" with calories every 12 weeks, Option 3 women may find it more helpful to follow their caloric intake on a daily basis. That doesn't mean obsessing about every calorie but staying within a general range of calories (sort of like sticking to a budget). Option 3 women include those who have some form of disordered eating, such as compulsive eating, who are more serious emotional eaters who can binge 1,000 calories or more at a sitting, or who—after years of the trials and torment of dieting—have lost touch with what fullness and satisfaction feel like. Option 3 also tends to suit women who mindlessly pick and snack their way through the day or who are on medications that can increase appetite and thus cause significant weight gain.

Not sure which option will work best for you? Pick the one that feels right and try it out. You can always try another. And regardless of which option you choose, fill in your Mind-Mouth-Muscle Daily Journal: Mouth (page 217) each day. Tracking your meals as well as your portions of Smart Proteins, Carbs, and Fats will keep you honest and reveal patterns in your eating behaviors, some of which may need tweaking.

It's all about flexibility. Today Option 2 may be your answer, but 2 years from now, you might want to give Option 1 a whirl. Be patient, and get comfortable with tweaking the system so that it works for you.

## Alternate Weight Removal Segment Formula

If you'd like, you can use this four-step formula for all Weight Removal Segments until you're ready to transition to the Maintenance Segment (which has its own formula; see page 228). You'll use your ever-changing resting metabolic rate, or RMR—the number of calories you burn while doing absolutely nothing—to determine the number of calories you must burn in that particular segment to ensure that you continue to remove weight.

The lighter you are, generally speaking, the lower your RMR, because a lighter body simply requires less energy to carry out its normal functions. So as you remove weight, your RMR will change. To continue to remove weight, you'll need to adjust your food and physical activity accordingly.

Although you don't have to use the formula below, I do think that doing it at least once every 12 weeks will raise your odds of making maximum progress. Do these calculations on paper and keep them with your Daily Progress Reports.

### 1. APPROXIMATE YOUR CURRENT RMR

Multiply your current weight by one of the RMR adjustment factors below. (See "Your Ideal Weight," page 142, to help you gauge.)

| If you're . . . | Multiply by . . . |
|---|---|
| 10–30 pounds overweight | 10 |
| 31–50 pounds overweight | 9 |
| 51 pounds or more overweight | 8 |

Your weight × RMR Adjustment Factor = ____ (Your RMR)

### 2. CALCULATE YOUR TOTAL CALORIES (TC)

Multiply your current weight by one of the physical activity factors below. For your first Weight Removal Segment *only,* multiply your RMR by your *current* level of physical activity rather than your *planned* level. After the first 12 weeks, if you've been working out regularly and developed more muscle, multiply by the activity level that reflects that current level of physical activity (PA).

- Sedentary (other than routine activities, no extra physical activity): 1.2
- Minimally active (20 to 30 minutes of nonintense physical activity one to three times a week): 1.3
- Moderately active (30 to 45 minutes of moderately intense physical activity five or more times a week): 1.4
- Very active (1 or more hours per day of intense physical activity): 1.7

Now, for your first Weight Removal Segment, multiply your RMR by your current level of physical activity:

RMR × PA= Total calories per day

Your TC: _____

## 3. DECIDE HOW MANY POUNDS YOU WANT TO REMOVE PER WEEK

Pick a realistic, weekly weight-loss goal from the options below, then subtract the number of calories indicated from your TC.

- To remove 0.5 pound a week, subtract 250 calories from your TC per day.
- To remove 1 pound a week, subtract 500 calories from your TC per day.
- To remove 1.5 pounds a week, subtract 750 calories from your TC per day.
- To remove 2 pounds a week, subtract 1,000 calories from your TC per day.

## 4. SPLIT YOUR WEIGHT-REMOVAL CALORIES BETWEEN HEALTHY EATING AND PHYSICAL ACTIVITY

I suggest a 50/50 split to start with, and here are examples of how to do it:

- To remove 0.5 pound a week, eat 125 calories less per day, move 125 calories more per day.
- To remove 1 pound a week, eat 250 calories less per day, move 250 calories more per day.
- To remove 1.5 pounds a week, eat 375 calories less per day, move 375 calories more per day.
- To remove 2 pounds a week, eat 500 calories less per day, move 500 calories more per day.

Try different combinations if you like. Just don't think you can achieve your goal by taking it all from Mouth or Muscle. Instead, you need to try to grab a little from each.

## Alternate Weight Maintenance Segment Formula

You weigh less, are a fitter woman now (you go, girl!), and your body's metabolic needs are quite different from when you started. This formula will help you figure out how much you can eat and how much you'll need to burn to maintain your current weight.

First, consult the BMI and body-fat charts (on pages 98 and 146) to see where your numbers fall. Then, follow these guidelines.

**If you're at goal weight and want to maintain it:** If you're within normal range in both the BMI and body-fat charts, simply multiply your weight by 10. Then, multiply that by your current level of physical activity. For example, if you were 170 pounds at the beginning of the program, and you've reached your goal weight of 135 pounds and are moderately physically active, your equation would look like this: $135 \times 10 = 1,350$.

Now, multiply 1,350 by your physical activity factor, 1.4: $1,350 \times 1.4 = 1,890$ calories. Voilà—your new RMR.

**If you're treading weight:** Multiply your current weight by the numbers in Step 2 of the Alternate Weight Removal Segment Formula (on page 226). In other words, if you're still 10 to 30 pounds overweight, multiply your current weight by 10. If you're 31 to 50 pounds overweight, multiply by 9. And if you're more than 50 pounds from your goal weight, multiply by 8. Then multiply that number by your *current* physical activity factor to get your new RMR.

My new RMR is : _____

Remember that these formulas are just starting points, and be prepared to fine-tune your program. If you gain weight despite following the guidelines, either reduce your food intake by 100 calories a day and/or increase your physical activity by 100 calories a day. Monitor your progress and be patient as your body adapts to its new weight, activity level, and way of eating. Remember, it was the tortoise who won the race, not the hare.

# Real-Life Success Stories

*Appendix E*

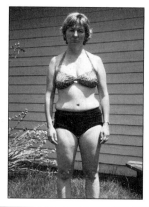 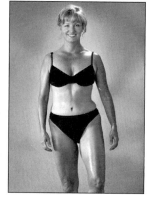 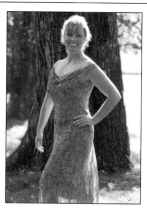

Before                    After                    2 Years Later

*"My son went off to college, and I got a new lease on life."*

I had plenty of excuses for not being fit and healthy. "Single parenting, self-employment, a crazy schedule, not enough time, don't know how, it's too hard. . . ." As a motivational speaker, life coach, and author, I supported and encouraged others but not myself. Hmm, something was wrong with this picture.

The day of my son's high school graduation, a fellow coach introduced me to the Challenge. Was I up for it? Reluctantly, I agreed. I didn't really know the scope of what I was committing to, but I sensed a milestone.

After seeing my "before" shots, I was fully committed, in a huge way. I couldn't fathom that the woman in those photos was me! My reluctance turned into determination and commitment, and I was up at 5:15 every day for the next 12 weeks to meet my "buddy coach" at the gym. With a month left to go, I proudly purchased a bikini for my "after" photo. The 18-year-old who sold me the bikini said, "Mama, if I was in that good shape, I'd show it off, too!" Sold! My best friend from childhood shrieked when she saw me, "You didn't look that good in high school!"

Ultimately, I lost 18 pounds, got down to 12 percent body fat, and went from a size 12 to a 6 or 8. I've kept my gains and get more powerful and resilient each day. I count the day I started in June as my "rebirthday."

My son went off to college, and Mom got a new lease on life not only with a new physique but with new confidence. My business has taken off, and I have extended my speaking and training to include Europe and Australia. I can now fly around the world, get off the plane, and my stamina ensures that I am ready to go. I am now fully committed to coaching other parents and kids in mental, emotional, and physical well-being. Because of this, I set the bar high for myself and plan to go the distance.

I no longer see myself as busy and overworked, as many of my friends do. I operate every day from the mindset of clarity, strength, and focus. I am *productive,* not overwhelmed. I cannot believe what this program has done for me and others like me.

*Diana Haskins*
*Age: 48*
*Personal Coach*
*Portland, Oregon*

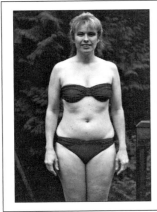 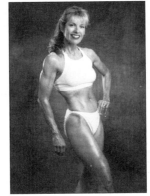 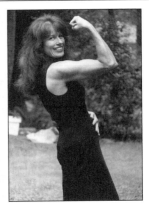

Before                    After                    4 Years Later

*"I stayed up all night reading about the Challenge—and my life changed forever."*

With a herniated disc, a cracked elbow, and bad knees—none of them from athletics—I was an unlikely participant in the Challenge. But I was almost 49 years old and was disgusted with my body. At 5 feet 10 inches and 176 pounds, I couldn't blame my size on being big-boned. I had elevated shopping for clothes that hid my rear end and thighs to an art form. I was also sleeping my life away because I was exhausted every minute of every day, working relentless hours managing two small businesses and doing volunteer work at my church.

One day, as I was walking past a magazine stand, a headline on the cover of a bodybuilding magazine jumped out at me. It said something about getting healthy and winning $100,000. That little tagline grabbed me enough to buy the magazine. That night, I read it from cover to cover. Within 24 hours, I had entered the Challenge and was standing on my deck in the rain while my husband, Peter, took my "before" picture.

The first day of the Challenge, I was up at 5:00 A.M. It was the first of many bleary-eyed days at the gym. I studied one exercise, performed it, and studied the next. I put up a huge chart in the kitchen to keep track of my weight loss and the exercise routines. My whole life got rearranged for the 84 days of the Challenge—everything revolved around it.

From the first week, I experienced more energy. By week 5, I couldn't get out of bed fast enough to see the changes in my body, which seemed to be occurring almost daily. The most wonderful thing was that Peter was watching my progress and making changes himself. Instead of living on sandwiches, he started filling his plate with vegetables, healthy carbs, and lean protein.

Twelve weeks later, I had lost 33 pounds, and 7 inches from my waist. I also made some changes in my personal life, such as slashing 50-hour workweeks to spend more time with my husband.

I still hit the treadmill four or five times a week and weights three or four times a week. I plan on being a 70-year-old hard-body! My life has changed unbelievably. My first book for women entrepreneurs was published, and a second is in the works. I now own an Internet business. None of that would have happened without the energy, confidence, and focus that I gained from my physical and mental transformation.

*Kristie Atkins*
*Age: 53*
*Business Owner*
*Woodinville, Washington*

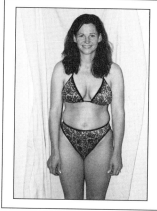 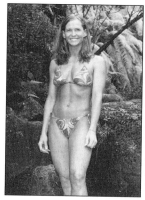 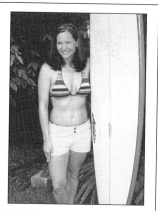

Before        After        3 Years Later

*"I learned that with hard work and self-love, you can change your life."*

For some time, I'd avoided replacing the battery in my scale. When I finally did, I was shocked: The display said I was carrying 157 pounds on my 5-foot-7 frame. I knew I'd been gaining weight, because my clothes were getting tighter by the day, but I didn't expect the number that stared back at me. My father died at 42 of a heart attack. I had heard about the Challenge, and I knew I was ready for a life change. I accepted the Challenge and was on my way.

When I took my "before" shots, I got my second shock—I really saw myself so different in the mirror from what the pictures showed. That was enough inspiration for me! My real inspirations, however, were my two boys, 2 and 4 years old. I wanted to see them graduate from high school, and to be a grandma someday. I wanted to see everything my father missed in his life.

My main obstacle was overcoming my craving for junk carbohydrates and chocolate. I had a bad habit of starving myself every day until 3:00 P.M., and then I would eat anything—and I mean anything. During those 12 weeks, I learned to feed my body, read the label on every food I put in my mouth. And my daily workout went from being a chore to being like food—I had to have it!

When the Challenge was over, I had gone from a size 10 or 12 to a size 3/4, from 28 percent body fat to 15 percent, and from 156 pounds to 130. I felt so great that I wanted to show the whole world the new me. My husband and I had planned a trip to Hawaii the week the Challenge was over. When I walked on the beach, I felt so proud and confident.

When I first looked at the before-and-after photos in the book, I thought, "There's no way a woman can change her body so drastically in 12 weeks!" Well, now I am one of them, and I have the pictures to prove it. I learned that with hard work and self-love, you can change your life. I will never forget that lesson.

*Michelle Cornell*
*Age: 34*
*Restaurant Manager*
*Roseville, California*

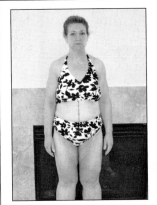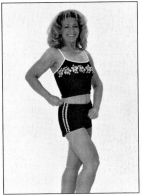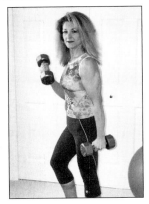

| Before | After | 1 Year Later |

*"After my surgery, the program helped me get into the best shape of my life."*

My life—and my weight—had long been out of control. At age 37, I was married, had two children, and weighed nearly 300 pounds.

I felt awful, mentally and physically. My feet, hips, and legs hurt constantly, I suffered from migraine headaches regularly, my marriage was on the rocks, and I was not able to play with my children. I felt that I would die if I did not get my weight under control. I came from a very unhealthy, overweight family. My mother developed breast cancer at 42, and my entire family had diabetes and high blood pressure. I knew my future was grim unless I did something soon.

In August 2002, I underwent gastric bypass surgery, and by January 2003, I had lost 105 pounds. At this time, I had been attending a local gym and doing cardio workouts. I noticed a trainer working with several women who had awesome bodies. I decided that I wanted to look like them. I made an appointment with the trainer, who did a light workout with me and mentioned the program.

I started the Challenge at 160 pounds and 30.3 percent body fat. Finding the time to exercise was difficult. I now had three children, one with special needs, and my marital problems caused me a lot of stress. I used that "stress energy" to work harder. My body and mind enjoyed the challenge of being pushed past previous limitations. I was not only surviving the Challenge; I was thriving!

I ended the Challenge at the end of June at 129 pounds and 15.8 percent body fat. My husband was impressed with my commitment, new attitude, and appearance, and I was able to play with my children for the first time. The look on my son's face when he asked me to play tag with him and I said "Yes" was priceless.

My self-confidence and energy are through the roof. I believe that I've made a difference in the lives of my children, whom I want to lead healthy lives; my parents; and my brother, who also accepted the Challenge and went from 465 pounds to 180 pounds. My transformation was one of the greatest accomplishments of my life.

*J. Renay Ternan*
*Age: 40*
*Hotel Sales Manager*
*Almont, Michigan*

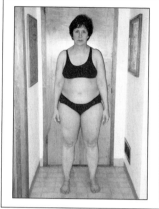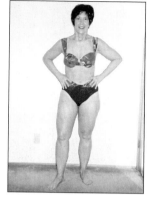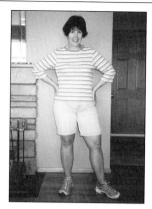

Before          After          2 Years Later

## *"Today I constantly look for new challenges, both physical and mental."*

At the time my "before" picture was taken, I thought I was in pretty good shape. I was running an hour almost every day and felt healthy enough, despite carrying some extra pounds. Also, I was blessed with a wonderful family, many friends, and a fulfilling career in teaching. Life was good!

So when I began the Challenge, I wasn't looking for major change. I figured I'd lose some weight, but I certainly did not expect any transformation. Was I ever wrong.

From day 1, I started changing. Ten minutes after I started my workout, I was dripping with sweat. Clearly, my body had been stuck in neutral for quite a few years. But when I started lifting weights and increasing the intensity of my aerobic workouts as part of the Challenge, my body woke up and took notice. And then the changes—both physical and mental—began.

I started paying attention to my diet for the first time in a long time. The weight loss now seemed effortless. I seemed to be eating more than ever before, and yet I started to drop 2 to 3 pounds each week. And I never felt hungry.

At the end of week 6, I suffered a back injury. For 3 days, I could barely walk, let alone work out. I wasn't sure I could continue the Challenge. But I kept to the eating plan and stayed positive by focusing on the progress I had already made. A week later, I returned to the gym.

At the end of 12 weeks, I was 28 pounds lighter and had dropped from a size 16 to a size 10. I lost 8 inches from my waist, 5 from my hips, and 3 from each thigh.

The mental transformation is harder to quantify. I started to see myself as an athlete. I gained confidence because I not only started the program but stayed with it for the entire 12 weeks. I can honestly say that nothing—nothing—has given me the feeling of empowerment that sticking to the Challenge did.

Today I constantly look for new challenges, both physical (sprint triathlons are my newest challenge) and mental (soon I will be pursuing a Ph.D.). In any case, life is good. Dare I say, awesome.

*Carol Coe*
*Age: 57*
*Teacher*
*Seattle, Washington*

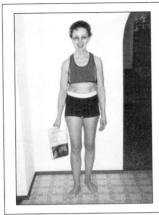 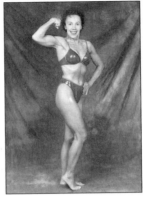 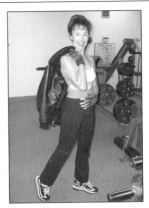

| Before | After | 3 Years Later |

## *"I want to break the mold for women over 50."*

I was fed up with my workout program. I'd been doing aerobics for 20 years, but my body never changed. I went to a local gym and told the trainer, Jana, I was tired of being like mush and wanted to "harden up." I went in for my first workout the next day.

I started with very light weights. When I wanted to increase the weight, Jana suggested that I get my bone density checked because she had noticed a curve in my spine. Imagine my shock when my doctor said that my bone density was 50 percent of what it should be! Because it's recommended that women with osteoporosis work out with free weights, my doctor was in favor of my continuing with the strength training. Then he prescribed medication, but I didn't fill the prescription. My diagnosis kept me determined to keep from becoming a stooped-over old lady before my time.

Jana was so impressed with my positive attitude, she suggested I enter the Challenge. I did some investigating, got inspired, and decided to go for it. I was so "pumped" that getting myself to the gym wasn't a problem. But eating six times a day was tough. I'd been eating only two meals a day because I thought more would cause weight gain. Instead, I ate all day (healthy food, of course), burned fat, and built muscle.

At the end of my Challenge, I'd reduced my body fat from 29.3 percent to 17 percent, and my weight from 127 pounds to 121 pounds. When I went for a checkup 6 months after my first visit, I had increased my bone density by 5 percent—without medication.

If you stop to think about it, it's a lot cheaper to go to a gym than to pay hospital bills or to lie around with broken bones. If you don't have your health, you don't have anything, and if you don't take care of yourself, nobody else is going to do it for you.

I want to break the mold for women over 50. If we don't step up to the plate, how are we going to know if we can hit the ball? No matter what the obstacle, be it your age or even a medical condition, keep sight of your goal. My intention is to use myself as an example to show it is never too late to start improving yourself.

*Lorinde Williams*
*Age: 63*
*Bakery Sales*
*Puyallup, Washington*

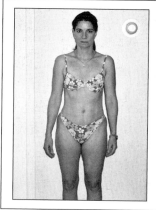
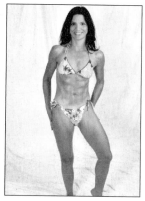
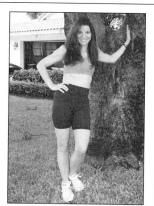

| Before | After | 2 Years Later |

*"I was a different person, not just on the outside but also on the inside."*

After 14 years of marriage and three kids, my body had changed. I wasn't severely overweight—in fact, I looked fine in clothes. But I didn't like how soft I'd become. I felt fat and unattractive and was dreading the big 4-0, which was only a few years away.

It was my sister who saved me. She started the Challenge, and 12 weeks later, this mother of three had completely transformed her body. I thought, "If she can do it with three kids, working full-time, so can I." I decided to enter the Challenge, too.

For me, the hardest part was making the time and commitment to get to the gym. Having always put my family's needs first, I was stingy with my "me" time. But now I was at the gym at 6:00 A.M. 6 days a week, then would rush home to get the kids off to school and get ready for work. (I'm a full-time emergency room nurse.)

The first 3 weeks were the most challenging. My body was constantly sore, and those early-morning gym sessions cut into my sleep a bit. Still, I pressed on, week after week. Before I knew it, the Challenge had become part of my life, as crucial to my life as breathing.

Week 9 was the turning point, and by week 12, I'd shrunk from a size 8 to a 1. My body fat percentage went from 20 percent to 13 percent. I was amazed at what I had achieved—I felt stronger and more powerful than ever before. I was a different person, not just on the outside but also on the inside. And despite my exhausting schedule, now I had the stamina to keep up with my hectic life.

I am proud of my body and my accomplishments, and I know I can conquer any mental and physical challenge that comes my way. Dedication and hard work have led me to strive toward lifelong fitness, and I've completed several 10-K runs and even a marathon. And my family life is great—my husband and I are like newlyweds, and I have the energy to keep up with my kids.

Don't let "I don't have time" be your excuse. You say you don't have time to give your body the care it needs? Yes, you do. If I can do it, anyone can!

*Ann Mon*
*Age: 42*
*Registered Nurse*
*Boca Raton, Florida*

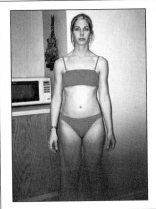 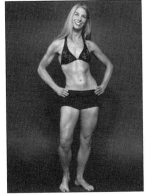 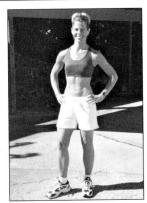

Before                           After                           1 Year Later

## *"Completing the Challenge has given me freedom."*

Seven years ago, I was diagnosed with an incurable and debilitating bladder disease called interstitial cystitis. Thankfully, after months of painful catheter treatments and mind-numbing drugs, I went into remission. Five years passed, with very minor flare-ups, until one day, almost overnight, the disease returned with a vengeance. I was devastated. Mentally and physically, I could not endure the catheter treatments and drugs again, so I began a quest to heal myself with alternative treatments. For months, it seemed, every waking moment was spent analyzing my body's reaction to everything: food, stress, sleep, air, water.

Eventually, I saw positive results—only to realize that I'd been so busy caring for my insides, I'd completely let my outsides go! I realized that I could never truly feel I'd beaten my disease unless my whole body was transformed. Around that time, my best friend entered the Challenge and his results were amazing, but deep in my heart, I felt I could never do it. After two failed attempts, I was proving myself right.

But one day as I lay on the sofa, recovering from a cold, a talk show host was speaking about defining moments. He said, "Life is made up of defining moments. . . . What are yours?" After mulling that over for a bit, I knew that the defining moments in my life were all de-

pressing hardships, and the most recent reflection of that was the return of my disease. How pathetic. Right then and there, I decided it was time to make a difference in my life. Once again, I readied myself for the Challenge.

This time, everything was different. Gone was my 7-year private pity party; in its place were determination and positive energy. Reading other people's success stories was like "Note to self: You are not the only one with problems." I threw myself into the Challenge and worked out every day, something I had not done since high school. I planned my meals every week and ate ultra-healthy, which was a challenge in itself. Little by little, I felt transformed, inside and out.

Completing the Challenge has given me freedom. No, my pain and disease haven't magically disappeared, but the barriers I placed in my head have. I'm free from the stipulations and obstacles chronically sick people place on themselves. The Challenge changed my life, and I can now proudly add completing it as one of the most positive defining moments in my life.

*Vicki Ewy*
*Age: 34*
*Executive Assistant*
*Liberty Lake, Washington*

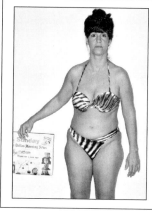 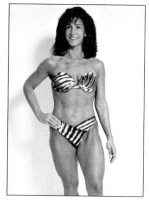 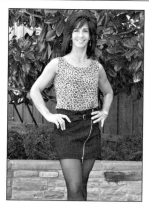

Before          After          4 Years Later

*"I transformed the core of my identity while I transformed my body."*

At 39, I married for the first time and started my own business. I'd always eaten under stress and was mortified to find myself in the grips of this destructive behavior once again. By the time I decided to enter the Challenge, I was at my all-time-high weight of 162 pounds. It was time to change!

Just after I entered the Challenge, an acquaintance sent me a picture of a female bodybuilder whose face strongly resembled mine, and to emphasize his point, he'd superimposed my name over hers. This photo became the center of my "dream board" of images that embodied my goals. Working with a trainer accelerated my pace.

I turned 40 in the 6th week of my program. I was physically pushing myself further than I ever had. But my biggest obstacles were internal. I had to remind myself to relax and trust that the program that had proved successful for so many others would work for me. When I started the Challenge, I said jokingly that the best indicator of my progress would be when strangers began to notice. This started to happen around week 7. But I had to laugh when someone I didn't know came up to me in the gym and said, "Excuse me, but are you the same person?" I was—just

smaller, yet more powerful. By week 12, I'd lost 27 pounds of fat and gained almost 4 pounds of muscle, and my body fat had dropped from 27.6 to 15.4 percent.

I was surprised at how emotional the Challenge was for me, and it wasn't until the end that I realized why: I had transformed the core of my identity while I transformed my body. The victory goes so deep within me. I am now free to move beyond the wall I created through doubt and fear. I have transformed the most destructive and limiting beliefs I held about myself and discovered parts of me I never knew existed.

Your belief that you can do it is most of the battle. Whatever I choose to put my hand to now, I know I can do it. I don't leave my self-care out of the equation, and it's a great feeling of freedom. My life is filled with great challenges and continuous successes, which used to be beyond my ability to even dream.

*Artemis Limpert-Decker*
*Age: 44*
*Business Development and Training*
*Richardson, Texas*

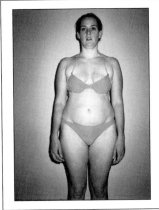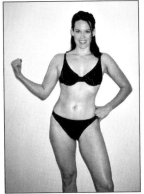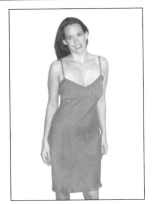

Before         After         1 Year Later

*"In a moment, you can make a choice that can change your life for the better."*

When you come close to losing someone, you begin to appreciate life like never before. In 2003, I heard news that my mother, who lives 3,000 miles away from me, had had a severe stroke. There was nothing I could do but hope for a miracle.

What happened to my mother was a wake-up call for me. A part of me had slipped away; I was overweight and unhappy, and I knew I had to take back my health. I knew that I did not want to settle for a life that was anything less but extraordinary. The next morning, I decided to enter the Challenge.

As a single mother with a demanding job, I have little time for myself. But the Challenge was a simple plan that fit into my busy schedule. My young son, then 18 months old, inspired me, too. Seeing him smile and copy me as I did my biceps curls kept me focused. I knew that each session was bringing me closer to my goal.

When I began the Challenge, I weighed 154 pounds. By the end, I had lost 27 pounds and dropped from a size 18 to a 6. My body fat now is 17 percent, and I have maintained my new weight. I feel stronger and have more energy than ever to keep up with my son, now 2.

I love the way I look, but nothing compares to the way I feel inside—empowered and alive. I now share my experience with others and try to inspire them to be the best they can be.

When I found myself, happiness and bliss found me. Every day is filled with miracles, and there is no reason to wait to feel this good about your life. In a moment, you can make a choice that can change your life for the better. Embrace it, dream it, and follow through. Set goals, and take the steps to achieve them, and you, too, will know what it feels like to be fully alive.

*Hollee Haas*
*Age: 32*
*Mother/Life Coach*
*Keizer, Oregon*

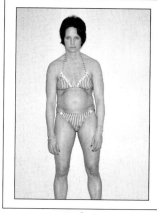 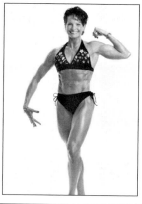 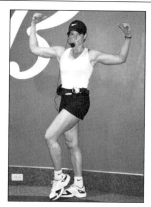

Before                          After                          1 Year Later

## *"The Challenge is a true testament to finding out what you are really made of."*

I completed the Challenge back in 1999 and was impressed with the results. But after I had my second child, I let myself fall back into bad habits and old patterns. I didn't like myself, the way I looked, or how I felt, physically or emotionally. And the excuses were getting old.

In 2003, I entered the Challenge again. I knew that this time I wasn't going to give anything less than 110 percent. Nothing was going to stand in my way.

I changed my nutrition and exercised every morning. Having quality time with my husband and two children is important to me, so my workouts had to happen very early—5:15 A.M. I just kept telling myself that I had to pay the price to reap the rewards.

I began the Challenge at a scale weight of 140 pounds and 24.8 percent body fat. Twelve weeks later, I was 132 pounds, and my body fat had dropped to 7.5 percent. All told, I lost 24.8 pounds of fat and gained 19.8 pounds of muscle.

I became addicted to this healthy way of life and have embraced fitness in a whole new light. Since I completed the Challenge, my life has never been better. I am strong—body, mind, and soul. I am now 38 years old, have two children, and consistently stay between 10 and 12 percent body fat. I can honestly say that I am in better shape now than I ever was before getting pregnant!

Because my progress was so remarkable, I wanted to help others change their lives as well. Everyone kept asking me what I was doing and why. I decided to try to find a way to help others on a daily basis. Now I'm a personal trainer and group exercise instructor for Bally Total Fitness. I continually help others to find their true selves and be the best that they can be through proper nutrition and exercise. The Challenge is a true testament to finding out what you are really made of and what is important to you.

When I reentered the Challenge, an amazing thing happened—I finally began to respect and love myself. Take the Challenge. You won't regret it.

*Maria Potvin*
*Age: 38*
*Group Fitness Instructor and Personal Trainer*
*North Canton, Ohio*

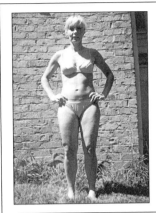
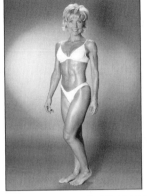
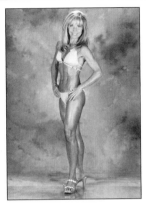

| Before | After | 4 Years Later |

*"Finally, I turned my excuses into* reasons *for completing the Challenge."*

My negative motivator for accepting the Challenge? Shopping for a swimsuit to hide my body and realizing I needed a wet suit. I was so depressed that I sent my husband out to buy me one. I felt unhappy, and my attitude affected my family. I was at the lowest point in my life.

That's when I saw the results the minister of my church, Jack, experienced during his 12-week transformation process. I was amazed. He changed not only his physique but his whole presence. He had a bounce in his step that wasn't there before. It was easy to see how proud he was when he shared his "before" and "after" pictures, and at that moment I knew I could feel that way, too. His excitement was contagious. I decided to accept the Challenge.

Believe it or not, in my "before" pictures I was starving myself and working out four or five times a week! I spent endless hours doing cardio, believing that it was the only way to keep my weight under control and slim down my ever-expanding thighs and behind. I fell for the myth that any kind of weight training would make me bulky. It's obvious that what I was doing wasn't working, yet I had tried every diet imaginable—I thought!

Life threw me more zingers than roses during the challenge. But I realized that what I once saw as an ob-

stacle was really only an excuse. I was the obstacle. Finally, I grabbed the bull by the horns, accepted responsibility, and turned all of my excuses into *reasons* for completing the Challenge.

I believe that the best testament to the effectiveness or success of the program is not the dramatic changes that occurred in my body after just 12 weeks, but that today, 4 years after completing my first Challenge, in addition to going from almost 20 percent body fat to 12.5 percent and losing 15 pounds, I lost almost 5 inches off each thigh and 4 inches off my behind, and I have kept it all off—with improvement!

The sense of pride that I got from successfully completing the Challenge is enormous. Those 12 weeks began a physical and emotional transformation that surpassed anything I could have dreamed. I could have never imagined "before" and "after" could be a time of such personal impact.

*Donna Szabo*
*Age: 45*
*Decorative Painter and Mother*
*Raleigh, North Carolina*

# Index

Underscored page references indicate boxed text and tables. **Boldface** references indicate illustrations and photographs.